crazy
sexy
juice

ALSO BY KRIS CARR

Crazy Sexy Love Notes (card deck)*

Crazy Sexy Kitchen: 150 Plant-Empowered Recipes to Ignite a Mouthwatering Revolution (with Chad Sarno)*

Crazy Sexy Diet: Eat Your Veggies, Ignite Your Spark, and Live Like You Mean It!

Crazy Sexy Cancer Tips

Crazy Sexy Cancer Survivor: More Rebellion and Fire for Your Healing Journey

*Available from Hay House

PLEASE VISIT:

Hay House USA: www.hayhouse.com®

Hay House Australia: www.hayhouse.com.au

Hay House UK: www.hayhouse.co.uk

Hay House India: www.hayhouse.co.in

crazy
sexy
juice

100+ simple juice, smoothie & nut milk recipes to supercharge your health

Kris Carr

FOOD PHOTOGRAPHY BY KATE LEWIS | COVER PHOTOGRAPHY BY BILL MILES

HAY HOUSE, INC.
Carlsbad, California • New York City
London • Sydney • Johannesburg
Vancouver • Hong Kong • New Delhi

Copyright © 2015 by Kris Carr

Published and distributed in the United States by: Hay House, Inc.: www
.hayhouse.com® • Published and distributed in Australia by: Hay House
Australia Pty. Ltd.: www.hayhouse.com.au • Published and distributed in
the United Kingdom by: Hay House UK, Ltd.: www.hayhouse.co.uk • Pub-
lished and distributed in the Republic of South Africa by: Hay House SA
(Pty), Ltd.: info@hayhouse.co.za • Distributed in Canada by: Raincoast
Books: www.raincoast.com • Published in India by: Hay House Publishers
India: www.hayhouse.co.in

INDEXER: Laura Ogar

Food photography © Kate Lewis 2015. Prop and food styling by Kate Lewis. Food
photography assistants: Melanie Buonavolonta & Devin Echle. Cover photo, page
11, 33, and 323 © Bill Miles. All other photos © Kris Carr

Library of Congress Cataloging-in-Publication Data

Carr, Kris.
Crazy sexy juice : 100+ simple juice,
smoothie & nut milk recipes to
supercharge your health / Kris Carr.
pages cm

ISBN 978-1-4019-4152-9 (hardback)

1. Body image. 2. Diet. 3. Nutrition.
4. Reducing diets. I. Title.

BF697.5.B63C357 2015

613.2'5--dc23

2015015287

10 9 8 7 6 5 4 3 2 1

1st edition, October 2015

Printed in the United States of America

DESIGN BY KARLA BAKER

FOR BUDDY AND LOLA,
my adopted fur children who give me
endless joy and remind me to add heaping
servings of wild fun to my life. And for
all of my wonderful readers, may you
love the skin you're in and be kind to
your precious selves.

Cheers to a long and vibrant life!

CONTENTS

welcome, gorgeous!

I am so happy you're joining me on this juicing and blending adventure. Get ready to be hooked on one of the healthiest habits around. *Crazy Sexy Juice* is your ultimate guide to the wonderful world of fruit and vegetable elixirs. The 100+ recipes in this book are over-the-moon delicious and nutritious, and range from fruity and refreshing summery potions to clean green healers, savory and spicy elixirs, creamy nut milks, and hearty superfood smoothies. If you're like me, it will be love at first sip!

No matter what stage of life we're in, we all want to feel awesome. We want to meet our full potential as we sail through our days with balance and ease. But many of us just don't know how to get there. In each of my books I've emphasized the importance of getting back to nature and the garden. Nature is the answer, dear friends. It has the power to restore and revitalize our bodies at the deepest level. A vibrant lifestyle doesn't have to be complicated, take a ton of time (and money), or add to your busy to-do list. You don't need to overhaul your kitchen or feel restricted. By simply adding these nutrient-dense beverages to your daily life, you'll be making health deposits (instead of withdrawals) and establishing a solid foundation for well-being. In fact, juicing and blending can be one of the easiest ways to achieve the freedom and vitality we seek.

Say hello to sustainable energy, glowing skin, and improved digestion. Say good-bye to inflammation, a lackluster appearance, and excess weight. Want to strengthen your immune system during cold season? Facing a health challenge and looking for a way to contribute to your well-being? Think of your green juices and smoothies as your personal pick-me-up in a glass.

We're gonna go deep because that's how I roll. I've left no stone unturned in this juicy manual for guzzling your way to glamorous (inside and out), and I can't wait for you to experience the goodness firsthand. I'll guide you through my handy tips and tricks learned over a decade of trial and triumph in the kitchen. In addition to expanding your kitchen repertoire with all the fabulous recipes in this book, you'll also get some serious brain food (AKA knowledge) so you can triumph on your own.

Here are a few of the topics we'll explore:

♡ The benefits and philosophy behind juicing and blending and the difference between the two. Plus, how to determine what's best for your lifestyle, schedule, and health needs

♡ How to create flavor combinations that tantalize your palate

♡ How to choose the best juicer, blender, and kitchen tools

♡ Ways to save money while prioritizing fresh, organic produce

♡ Suggestions for juicing and blending on the go

♡ Troubleshooting advice for common kitchen mishaps

♡ Tips for selection, storage, and preparation of the ingredients found in this book

♡ Top nutrients and health benefits of your produce, superfoods, and other ingredients

♡ Answers to frequently asked questions and health concerns

♡ Self-care hints to nurture your body and soul

♡ Tips on how to get your family on board and make this lifestyle stick

♡ And so much more . . .

If you're interested in reconnecting to your body and reinvigorating your system, I've included an easy and energizing three-day cleanse toward the end of the book. This plan is for everyone: folks who are just getting started with juices and smoothies, juicing and blending pros, and those of you who love the taste of these drinks but sometimes find it challenging to stick with the habit.

Junk and convenience foods seduce us all. Giving ourselves a healthy reboot (AKA cleanse) can bring us back to center and sanity. Think of it as an opportunity to reset your digestion and polish the already magnificent diamond that is you! This cleanse isn't about starvation, deprivation, or calorie counting: it's about recalibrating our palates and renewing our bodies by introducing cleaner, healthier foods into our lives.

During the three-day cleanse you'll enjoy a variety of delicious juices, smoothies, nut milks, and, yes, actual food that's both nourishing and satisfying—because we all love to chew. I don't know about you, but I get "hangry" (AKA hungry and angry) when my belly grumbles.

Simple steps can lead to profound change. One sip at a time, you can improve your life and your family's lives. It's happened to me and it can happen to you. When I first started sharing my journey online, I was amazed at the feedback and testimonials that came in as my story and teachings grew in popularity. Today, thousands of people have embraced the healthy habits I write about, and the results have been both heartwarming and remarkable. Reducing inflammation, healing chronic conditions, getting off excess medications, breaking free from the aches and pains that diminish our quality of life—the list grows by the day. The best part? People have been getting their joy back. What started as a tiny blog has turned into a hub of health and happiness with over a million readers every month. Sometimes I wish I could go back in time and tell my younger self that it would all be okay. Yet, at my darkest hour, I probably wouldn't have listened.

My Crazy Sexy Story

Like some of you, I found these healthy lifestyle practices when I was in a personal crisis. Isn't that how so many transformations occur? We get knocked to our knees and decide to look for a better way. If you've been a part of my community for a while, then you probably know my story. In case you don't, here's the Cliffs Notes version: On Valentine's Day of 2003, I was diagnosed with a rare and incurable (yet thankfully slow-growing) stage IV cancer.

I was scared and didn't know where to turn. Living with an incurable disease can feel very disempowering, like there's nothing you can do to make your life better. After considerable depression, I pulled myself up by my bootstraps and took action. For years I had been feeling like garbage—I was sick, tired, and emotionally stuck. I struggled with disordered eating and low self-esteem. Basically, I didn't value myself very much, and I certainly didn't know what to eat or drink or how to deal with the toxic emotions and limiting beliefs that were holding me back.

For me, cancer put everything into focus. It helped me stop putting off a brighter day and a better tomorrow. If I couldn't be cured, could I still be healthy? Could I feel good in the skin I'm in, regardless of my medical condition? Could my heart be filled with joy and gratitude for my life and the world around me even though my plans had taken a drastic connection between my health, the earth, and all its beings. And that, my friends, has kept me true to caring for the world and myself each and every day. It's the backbone of my wellness practice, and I'm eternally grateful to have discovered and embraced this ritual with my whole heart.

If you've read some of my previous books, including *Crazy Sexy Cancer Tips, Crazy Sexy Diet,* and *Crazy Sexy Kitchen,* then you know that my diet is plant-based, which means it's loaded with a whole lot of greens, vegetables, fruits, nuts, seeds, legumes, and whole grains. Adjusting to a new way of eating takes motivation and a willingness to experience new tastes, textures, and flavor combinations. But if you're looking to start with a single dietary improvement, juicing and blending take the cake (so to speak).

I'm excited to share these practices with you. While this book isn't meant to be a cure-all, or a replacement for medical advice or care, it is a manifesto of juicy wisdom gathered from years of research and experience. Let the benefits of these blends speak for themselves. You'll be so glad you gave them a whirl!

It's been more than a decade since my diagnosis and I continue to live a joyful, healthy life with a chronic disease. If I can do that, just think of what *you* can do!

Are you ready to dive in? Excellent! I hope you experience juicing and blending just the way I have: as an easy and delicious journey into the transformative powers of fresh, raw fruits and vegetables. Slap on an apron and let's have some fun, hot stuff!

turn? The answer was a full-blown, Technicolor HECK YES. Suddenly I felt excited. Why wait? Live now. Love now. Go for it.

That pivotal decision kicked off my own personal wellness revolution. It brought me back to nature and closer to the people and animals I love so much. If you'd asked me to drink my greens in my 20s, I would've said no thanks, and reached for a martini instead. Let's be real—my biggest connection to chlorophyll was the potted spider plant sitting in the window of my New York City apartment.

Cut to today, years after I took off for Upstate New York, armed with a juicer, a blender, and a big ole bag of greens. My juices and smoothies continue to be a big part of my daily wellness practice. This simple habit—buying or growing vegetables, washing, prepping, and creating my elixir of the day—keeps me nourished and energized. It's been my gateway to truly feeling that

getting ready
for health

1

BENEFITS AND PHILOSOPHY

Mom said it best:
"Eat your vegetables!"

It's the first commandment of healthy eating, yet chowing down on fruits and veggies seems to be the suggestion that Americans struggle with most. The latest dietary guidelines call for a minimum of 2½ to 6½ cups of fruits and vegetables per day. Yet a 2010 study showed that only about 25 percent of U.S. adults meet those daily requirements (unless you count ketchup and fries). For adolescents it's even worse. Sadly, we're doing a lousy job with our fruits and veggies, and it's taking a toll on our precious health.

Fruit and vegetable consumption is associated with reduced rates of heart disease, high blood pressure, and some cancers. It's also associated with less bodily inflammation (we'll get to that soon), less stress, better immunity, and leaner weight. With our less-than-ideal fruit and veggie noshing, it's no surprise that America is leading the way with obesity, heart disease, type II diabetes, cancer, and a huge number of other chronic diseases. We're skimping on the foods that help us stay healthy and strong, while loading up on the stuff that makes us sick. And besides the impact on individuals, this way of eating has created an unsustainable crisis for the country as a whole.

As a self-proclaimed plant pusher, I'd love nothing more than to tell you that it's a breeze to prepare fresh fruits and veggies each and every miraculous day. In my ideal world, we would all have personal nannies and endless hours to have fun and take care of ourselves. But that's just not often the case. Fruits and vegetables do require some extra time and elbow grease for washing, peeling, and chopping. They also don't keep as long as processed foods and aren't as easy to travel with—cue the packaged stuff. We don't have to think about it—just open the box or bag and we're good to go, go, go.

And let's be honest, in most cases processed food is cheaper. Or at least it seems that way while standing in the checkout line. But the truth is that the actual price of bad food is much higher once you consider the health-care costs and the environmental impact. Unfortunately, government policies make it really hard for fruits and veggies to compete. Our tax dollars go toward subsidizing only a few major mega-crops, like corn (you guessed it, corn syrup!) to keep their prices low. So until broccoli can afford a lobbyist, the 99-cent happy (crappy) meal will rule for too many people.

I believe another important reason folks don't eat enough fruits and veggies is because they haven't experienced the taste of fresh, ripe produce. Try eating a just-picked tomato from a garden and compare it to the flavorless cardboard version from the supermarket. Bleh!

It's also about the way they're cooked. Many of us haven't been exposed to the full culinary wow-factor of plants. For some, scary childhood memories of Mom's mushy, overcooked broccoli tarnish its appeal. I'm pretty certain that if we could all taste vegetables that were prepared well, we'd fall deeply-madly in love with them. Watching the response to *Crazy Sexy Kitchen* is proof positive of this! But suppose you don't have much time or don't even like cooking. Suppose you don't have many resources. Suppose you've been traumatized by a nasty dish of gray lima beans. How on earth do you develop a taste for fruits, vegetables, and greens?

The answer to these questions lies within the pages of this book. It resides in these delicious, colorful, produce-packed drinks. Creative juice and smoothie combinations can taste absolutely incredible. They're a perfect way to persuade veggie-phobes to eat more produce. Plus, they're jam-packed with good stuff. Get this: it can take over a pound of fruits and vegetables to make one juice. An average green juice at Casa Carr includes a half head of romaine, a big fistful of kale, two cucumbers, a couple of green apples, lots of lemon, and a few stalks of celery. That's a lot of produce (and nourishment), and there's no way I could sit down and nosh it all at once. Run it through a juicer, though, and you have a supremely healthy (not to mention delicious) daily habit. The same goes for blending. When you're on the go, is it always realistic to sit and eat a banana, a cucumber, avocado, kale, and coconut water? Probably not—but put them all together in a quick smoothie and you've got yourself a meal.

So, if you're making an effort to flood your diet with fresh, nutrient-dense, hydrat-

ing produce, juices and smoothies are going to be your new best friends. Now let's chat about some of the incredible health benefits they offer you.

pH: A pHabulous Guide

You'll notice me talking about "acid" and "alkaline" throughout the book. What exactly am I referring to?

The quality of our inner ecology will determine our overall health. Life is more connected than we think. Everything from the cells in our bodies to the life in the oceans is affected by pH. The term *pH* stands for "potential hydrogen" and really just means the level of acidity or alkalinity of a given substance. To get technical, pH measures the hydrogen ions in a particular solution. Solutions that contain a lot of free hydrogen ions are considered to be acidic, while fewer ions means alkaline. In our case, that "solution" refers to our body's fluids, tissues, and organs.

As with most health-related barometers, pH is all about balance. The chemistry of your body's fluids and tissues can be measured on a pH scale of 0 to 14. Seven on the pH scale is neutral. Less than 7 is considered acidic, and greater than 7 is alkaline. Our cells are happy, healthy, and at their peak performance when living in a slightly alkaline environment. Because of that, our bodies hover in the 7.365 to 7.45 range. Even the slightest dip or rise in pH can have disastrous consequences, so our bodies are programmed to maintain that slightly alkaline threshold of 7.365 no matter what—it's basically set in stone.

Here's the potential rub: the standard American diet (SAD) is filled with acidic foods and substances, including dairy, meat, highly processed food products, and refined sugar, not to mention environmental toxins. Some research suggests that, in order to keep your pH in balance, your body will have to work harder to neutralize the acidic load, which can result in a gradual degeneration of health. Other research claims that our diets don't matter because the body will correct itself without cost to our health. So what's true? Who knows—the jury is still out. But we do know that kidney stones and gout are associated with high acid diets, so obviously there's something to pH and

food. So why not tip the scale in the alkaline direction?

The easiest way to do that is to minimize the overly acid-forming offenders (refined sugars and grains, processed foods, dairy, meat) and to maximize alkaline-forming, mineral-rich foods. These include dark leafy greens, wheatgrass, veggies, green juices, smoothies, and certain grains. Eating these goodies will flood our bodies with alkalinity and a hefty dose of vitamins and other micronutrients.

Do we have to eat alkaline foods 100 percent of the time? No way, and that's actually not possible for good health. Don't think of it as good and bad or black and white. There are definitely shades of gray. Some foods that are slightly acidic, like beans, grains, and nuts, are essential for proper nutrition on a plant-powered diet. Again, it's the *highly* acidic foods that we should limit as much as possible. Plus, life wouldn't be as fun without the occasional morning joe or slice of birthday cake. Overall, our goal is to make more energy deposits than withdrawals. Our bodies forgive the detours and exploration, as long as they don't take place 24-7.

Taming the Flames: Inflammation

Inflammation is a hot topic that's often written about online and in magazines. While it can certainly damage our health, inflamma-

tion is actually a normal part of our body's defense system against injury or attack. The swelling and redness you get around a cut, for example? That's inflammation at work. The swelling is an attempt to isolate pesky bacteria and prevent infection. The release of histamines, which are commonly associated with allergies, is another example of an inflammatory reaction. In this case, the histamines help to dilate blood vessels, which allows our white blood cells to reach and destroy bacteria, allergens, and other microscopic particles that cramp our style.

Clearly, inflammation is necessary and vital to our well-being. But the problem arises when improper diet and lifestyle choices cause it to run amok. Instead of serving as a natural response to trauma, injury, or infection, it takes up permanent residence in our bodies, wreaking havoc on our health. Chronic pain, allergies, hay fever, atherosclerosis (AKA hardening of the arteries—often a precursor to heart disease), and even some cancers are associated with chronic inflammation. Inflammation can also show up along with other health conditions, like autoimmune diseases.

While chronic and systemic inflammation can be tricky to manage, certain positive lifestyle practices are very effective in helping tame it. Stress reduction is at the top of the list. Stress, along with long-term depression and anxiety, is associated with higher levels of inflammatory response. Meditation, positive affirmations, walks with friends, reading, laughing, sleeping or napping, painting,

journaling, singing, shaking your booty—all of these activities help tame the flames that bring us down. Exercise and adequate sleep are especially critical, as is weight management. Weight gain and excess body fat can signal a crisis to your system, throwing inflammatory responses into high gear.

Diet can be your best ally in turning off inflammation. Foods can either stoke or fight the fires of systemic inflammation. Foods that contribute to inflammation include (you guessed it!) refined sugars, processed grains, junk food, meat, and dairy—not surprisingly, the very same foods that fall on the acidic side of the pH scale. See a pattern here?

Meanwhile, the same foods that can help to keep our pH balance healthy and flood our body with nutrients are also our best allies in the fight against systemic inflammation. Fruits and vegetables—especially dark, leafy greens—are some of the most potent anti-inflammatory agents known. The more of them you eat, the more you'll be able to switch your inflammatory response to the "off" position, resulting in a better quality of life. If you're dealing with a health condition that's linked to chronic inflammation—such as autoimmune diseases, arthritis, allergies, or heart disease—then this is the perfect time for you to be immersing yourself in the exciting world of green drinks. Other plant-based inflammation fighters include sweet potatoes, olive oil, walnuts, flax, certain spices, and organic soy.

Powerful Prevention: Phytonutrients

Think of phytonutrients as your personal bodyguards against free radicals and diseases that threaten your health on a daily basis. Phytonutrients give plant foods (and only plant foods: you can't find them in animal products) their show-stopping colors. These natural chemicals have been associated with better eye health, immunity, and prevention of a host of different types of cancer. (Yay!)

Here are just a few notable phytonutrients:

♡ ANTHOCYANINS—compounds that create blue, purple, and red hues in foods like eggplants, blueberries, cherries, red onions, and grapes—have been associated with reduced risk of cardiovascular disease.

♡ CAROTENOIDS give veggies red, orange, and yellow hues. They're associated with eye health (if you ever wondered why you've been told to munch on carrots for better vision) and are antiaging. Find them in peppers, carrots, and winter squash.

♡ ELLAGIC ACID, found in berries and pomegranates, may help to slow the growth of cancer cells. It may even help your liver to neutralize cancer-promoting compounds.

♡ GLUCOSINOLATES, found in cruciferous veggies, may be potent cancer fighters.

♡ HESPERIDIN, found in citrus fruits, has been shown to help reduce inflammation.

♡ LUTEIN—found in green, leafy vegetables like spinach, kale, and collards—helps to prevent eye diseases, including cataracts and macular degeneration.

♡ LYCOPENE, associated with red and pink fruits and vegetables, may lower the risk of prostate cancer. You'll find it in tomatoes, watermelon, and grapefruit.

♡ PHYTOESTROGENS—found in soy foods, flax seeds, and sesame seeds—mimic the effect of estrogen very mildly in the body. They've been shown to help with menopause, and they're also associated with a reduced risk of bone loss and a reduced risk of cancer.

♡ QUERCETIN—found in apples, berries, kale, and onions—may help reduce people's risk of asthma.

♡ RESVERATROL, found in purple-stained fruits and vegetables (blueberries, grapes), is anti-inflammatory, and it's even been associated with life extension in certain studies.

The list goes on, but you get the bright idea: you want these incredible, potent compounds in your belly. And you guessed it again—juices and smoothies are a perfect vehicle. If you want to know more about which fruits and vegetables are particularly rich in phyto-goodness, check out the list of superstar ingredients starting on page 65.

Hydration and Elimination

Did you know that approximately 63 million people in North America are constipated? Ouch! One study puts the prevalence at 27 percent of our population. That's a lot of backed-up and cranky folks, and we all know what that feels like: headachy, bloated, and uncomfortable.

The war on a stagnant pooper has to be waged on two fronts. First, we need more fiber. Like phytonutrients, fiber is found only in plant foods. Because we can't actually digest fiber, it passes right through us, taking all sorts of nasty debris with it, including harmful bacteria, excess cholesterol, and stagnant waste. (Pee-ew!) Consuming dietary fiber is associated with a strong immune system, a healthy balance of gut bacteria, reduced cholesterol, and a reduced

risk of heart disease. Fiber also helps control the way our bodies use sugar, which keeps appetite and blood sugar in check (and helps prevent blood sugar–related illnesses like metabolic syndrome and type II diabetes). Perhaps most important, we can't keep our elimination moving without the stuff. Low-fiber diet? A stopped-up system.

Thanks to the vegetable deficit we've already touched on, the average American gets only half of his or her recommended daily dose of fiber. (No wonder we can't go!) The solution is simple: eat (and drink) more plants; poop more.

Keep in mind that when we eat lots of healthy fiber, we also have to increase our consumption of water. Think of fiber as the stuff that helps bulk up your BMs; water is what helps keep the trains moving. One of the overlooked benefits of fruits and vegetables is that they're incredibly hydrating (unlike refined carbs and meat and processed junk, which actually dehydrate us). Getting more fruits and vegetables—especially in juice or smoothie form—can help keep our systems flooded with hydration. And drinking water throughout the course of your day is an important and easy habit. Even if you're loading up on smoothies and juices, you still need some garden-variety H_2O to keep things moving!

Sugar

How many times have you heard a friend, colleague, or neighbor complain about a sweet tooth? The fact is, more and more people are struggling with sugar addictions these days, and it's easy to see why. Americans eat *a lot* of sugar—over 150 pounds of *added* sugar per person, per year. Try hauling that around in your Halloween bag!

The American Heart Association recommends that we get no more than half of our discretionary calories (AKA extra calories our bodies don't need to function) from added sugars. This comes to about 26 to 32 grams of added sugar per person, per day, or about 6 to 8 teaspoons of added sugar. Sadly, the vast majority of Americans exceed the AHA's guideline significantly.

I've said it before and I'll say it again: you are sweet enough, darling. Consuming too much sugar (especially the processed stuff) isn't self-loving or nurturing. In fact, it can add up to some pretty serious medical life lemons. Excessive sugar consumption is associated with obesity, metabolic syndrome, heart disease, type II diabetes, and cancer. To make matters worse, it's nearly impossible to avoid in the grocery aisles. Sugar—which you may also see labeled as sucrose, maltose, corn syrup, malt syrup, dextrose, maltodextrin, high fructose corn syrup, or glucose solids—hides in nearly all processed foods, from pizza to salad dressing to spaghetti sauce to lunch meats. It's our favorite food additive, and it may be our most addictive . . . and deadly.

But here's the good news: you can take charge of your health and help protest the overabundance of sugar in our food system by becoming a more sugar-savvy consumer.

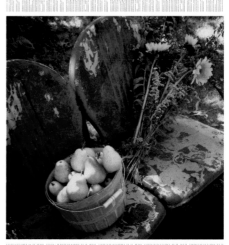

Begin by doing more of your own cooking, so you can avoid all the sugar-laden products and processed foods that fill our grocery stores. Start to cut back on added sugars (table sugar, corn syrup, malt syrup, sucrose, and artificial sweeteners) as much as possible. Finally, learn to satisfy your sweet cravings with fruits and vegetables, which are nature's own perfect sweets.

It's important to understand that all sugar is not created equal. One response to the sugar epidemic is to deem *all* sugars off-limits, but there's a big difference between natural sugars and added sugars. The reason that government agencies and health experts make a point of discouraging "added sugars" is because these types of sugars are heavily processed and devoid of any natural nutrients. They bring our blood sugar up without supplying our bodies with anything healthful: a lose-lose situation.

Naturally occurring sugars, on the other hand—I'm talking about the sugars in fresh fruits and vegetables—deliver sweetness while also providing vitamins, minerals, and concentrated stores of powerhouse phytonutrients. The sugars in fruit (or sweeter vegetables, like carrots, beets, and sweet potatoes) also come packaged with fiber, which helps us feel full and slows the absorption of sugar into our bloodstream. Plus, the micronutrients in fresh fruit may prevent the uptake of sugar in our small intestine. This means that we can enjoy the delightful sweetness and health benefits of fresh fruit without having to worry about mood-busting highs and lows and blood sugar spikes. Not surprisingly, evidence shows that populations who eat more fruit have a lower BMI and lower risk of developing many chronic diseases, including high blood pressure, heart disease, stroke, certain cancers, type II diabetes, digestive diseases, and obesity.

Of course, if you have special reason to be vigilant about the amount of sugar in your diet—for example, if you're a cancer patient or you have diabetes—then you may want to exercise some mindfulness even with naturally occurring sugars. For you, it may be wise to seek out fruits that are lower in sugar, and to use only moderate amounts of fruit and sweet veggies in your green drinks. A lot of juice and smoothie recipes out there are on the supersweet side of the spectrum, and with that in mind, I give you a range of options and plenty of resources for taking control of the sweetness of your green

elixirs. On page 49, you'll find my tips for balancing fruits and veggies in your juices and smoothies, along with some pointers on how to reduce the sugar in any recipe you love. Finally, I'll teach you all about the glycemic index and glycemic load, measurement systems that can help you to figure out which fruits are more suitable for you and your health needs.

Fats & Protein

We need good quality fats and protein to thrive and, luckily, the plant kingdom provides them in abundance. Essential fatty acids (omega 3, 6, and 9) are necessary for your nervous system, your immune function, and your reproductive and cardiovascular systems. They also play a vital role in cell membrane function and formation, allowing nutrients and oxygen to be absorbed and waste to be excreted.

Most fruits and veggies contain trace amounts of these fatty acids. Others, like coconut, avocado, hemp, flax, and raw nuts and seeds contain an abundant amount of these life-sustaining nutrients. The days of being scared of fat are long over. We now know that fat is a crucial component to a healthy diet, and you'll find a well-proportioned amount of it in these recipes, especially the smoothies.

Protein helps build and repair tissues. It's used to make hormones and enzymes and is important for cell function. Your gorgeous hair and nails are basically made of protein.

But although we can't function without it, many people are getting more protein than they actually need, and from poor quality sources like factory-farmed meats.

Contrary to popular belief, animal products aren't the only source of protein. Nuts, nut milks, avocado, and even leafy greens are all great sources too. In fact, hemp and chia seeds are considered complete sources of protein. If you regularly include these ingredients along with beans and grains in your diet, you'll be doing a great job at meeting your body's need for protein.

Another benefit of healthy fats and proteins is that they keep you fuller and more satisfied longer. They also help slow down the absorption of sugar into your bloodstream, thus minimizing insulin spikes that tax your system.

Now that you've brushed up on some basic nutrition nuggets, let's get the skinny on juicing and blending, what appliances you'll need, how to craft a perfect elixir on your own, and other handy tips. Knowledge is power in life and in the kitchen. By the time you're done reading this book and exploring these recipes, you'll be a wealth of wisdom and a fountain of youth.

NUT BUTTER

When buying nut butters, do your best to keep them raw. When nuts are roasted using high heat, the oils are damaged and can often go rancid. Also, avoid products with added sugars (especially the fake stuff).

2

JUICING AND BLENDING, DEMYSTIFIED

What's the difference between juicing and blending? If I had a buck for every time someone asked me that question, I'd be able to stock your fridge with organic produce for life. Each method has its unique perks, but rest assured they're both fabulous ways to incorporate nutrition-packed produce into your diet.

Juicing extracts the liquid from the fruits and vegetables, leaving the fiber behind. By removing the fiber, all of the nutrients in the plant's juice—vitamins, minerals, enzymes—instantly flood our bodies with goodness. Just think of the added volume of veggies you can pack in your belly, sweet unicorns! Even those of us with the heartiest of appetites would find it challenging to consume the same amount of raw vegetables and fruits with a fork.

Juicing also gives your digestive system a little rest, and since your body works hard on your behalf 24-7, it's nice to give it some R&R. "But I thought fiber was good for you?" Yes, beautiful, you're right. And if you're upgrading your overall diet to include whole foods, you'll be getting plenty of it—especially if you include smoothies and healthy, home-cooked chow. My books *Crazy Sexy Kitchen* and *Crazy Sexy Diet* are great primers if you need more of a plan (and mouthwatering recipes).

Got digestive ouchies? Juicing is a great option for folks who love to eat plant-rich diets but whose digestive systems are too sensitive to handle lots of fiber. If that's you, juicing ensures you can enjoy the benefits of boatloads of awesome produce without suffering any tummy troubles for your efforts. For people focused on healing or repair in general, juices offer maximum health benefits in a gentle, easy-to-digest, easy-to-assimilate form.

Blending on the other hand . . . blends! The ingredients are whirled and pureed into scrumptious smoothies, fiber and all, providing the benefits of fruits and veggies along with their heart-healthy, gut-friendly fiber.

Folks who are watching their blood sugar sometimes prefer blending to juicing because the fiber ensures a slow and steady absorption of sugar into your bloodstream. It's definitely possible to create juice blends that are lower in sugar (for more information, turn to page 53), but if you feel that smoothies are a more appropriate option for you, that's fine. The important thing is to get green drinks in your diet. Take your time and experiment with both juices and smoothies to discover which one or what combination of the two is right for you and your health needs. In a typical week, my morning concoctions are usually split about 50/50 between juicing and blending. But it's not a hard and fast rule; I go with my "gut," so to speak.

Besides all the great fiber, smoothies allow you to use fantastic foods that would piss your juicer off. Take sprouts, for instance, those tiny powerhouses of plant nutrition. Sprouts will shoot right through a centrifugal juicer without getting juiced, but they blend up perfectly in smoothies. Nut butters and superfood powders can give you (and your energy levels) a powerful boost, but they can't be juiced. Blend them up, though, and you're on your way to all sorts of unusual, flavorful, and even medicinal drinks. (See page 195 for some of my favorite health-lifting smoothie formulas.)

Smoothies have another important advantage, which is that they can help you feel fuller longer. Protein, healthy fats, and carbs create sustainable energy. If you fill up your smoothies with lots of nutrient-packed ingredients, they can even serve as well-rounded, convenient, and delectable meals.

Did I mention snacks? Smoothies can work as an afternoon snack or a refreshing sip on a sizzling summer day. The fun thing about smoothies is that you can choose your own adventure: add healthy fat and protein for a meal or postworkout-worthy treat, or keep things light for a midmorning revitalizer.

Smoothies are also a great way to sneak veggies into finicky kids' meals, or to help your family (or yourself) develop a taste for leafy greens. Yet another great advantage to blending is time. Blending is faster than juicing, without a question, and the cleanup is a snap, too.

The bottom line is that both juicing and blending are wonderful and efficient ways to maximize your consumption of the good stuff: greens, vegetables, fruits, and superfoods. One has fiber, the other doesn't. One allows for maximal nutrient intake in one sitting, while the other allows you to incorporate a wide range of ingredients and take advantage of fiber, protein, and healthy fats. Over time, you'll probably find yourself enjoying both types of drinks according to your schedule, appetite, and mood, and that's great—it's hard to go wrong when you're flooding your body with alkaline goodness! Choose what makes you happy and motivated to drink your way to wellness.

Now, let's dive a little deeper into the juicing and blending processes.

All About Juicing

So here you are at the start of your juicing journey. You're probably wondering what juicer you'll need, how to create juices that

are as delicious as they are healthful, and how to prep and store your juice so that it's as fresh as possible. I've got you covered. But before we jump into that, let's talk schedule.

A lot of people ask me what the best time of day to juice is. My answer: Whatever time works for you, tootsie! There are no rules; it all depends on your schedule and lifestyle. But there are some ways to create a routine that fits your rhythms.

Morning is my favorite time to juice because it starts my day off with a boost of alkaline, plant-powered nourishment. It also gives me energy and helps me resist the lure of coffee—a less nourishing, more acidic way to kick off the day (though I do worship a good cup o' joe from time to time).

If mornings are too hectic for you (kids, partners, dogs, ponies), and you're able to take an afternoon break, then make that your ritual. Afternoons are an excellent time to sip some plant-powered goodness, especially if you find yourself hunting down sugary snacks when the 2 to 4 P.M. energy slump hits. A yummy juice will curb your enthusiasm for a donut, put some pep in your step, and blow away brain fog until din-nertime.

If you come home from work and find yourself immediately reaching for that bottle of Chardonnay and a bag of chips, then make a green juice and sip on it as you prep dinner. Pour it into a lavish cocktail glass, as I do. Presentation also helps lift the mood, darling.

If all else fails, consider investing in the type of juicer that allows you to prep your morning juice one night in advance (don't worry . . . I'll explain), and then sip it on the way to work.

Choosing a Juicer

There are plenty of green machines on the market to satisfy any budget, although the cheapest ones may not always make you happiest. Think of your juicer purchase as an investment in your long-term wellness, energy, and radiance. We want to squeeze every possible ounce of goodness into our glasses. Unfortunately, crappy juicers can produce crappy yield. If you're going to spend money on high-quality, organic fruits and vegetables, and time preparing them for juicing, you might as well be sure that the machine you use helps maximize their nutrients and power.

In general, there are two main categories of juicers for noncommercial use. I'll explain them more thoroughly in a moment, but the basic difference is that one works quickly and is easy to clean but isn't necessarily top-of-the-line when it comes to the longevity of your juices. The other creates juices that may contain more nutrients and enzymes and can keep for a few days, but takes more time and can be harder to clean than its quicker counterparts.

Frankly, the choice you make depends on your goals and your lifestyle. If you're a hard-core raw foodie who wants to invest in a killer

WHEATGRASS

Wheatgrass gets an Olympic gold medal in health. Widely acclaimed for its nutritional and therapeutic properties, wheatgrass is teeming with phytonutrients—specifically antioxidants, which help keep aging and degeneration at bay. Wheatgrass may help protect the liver against alcohol damage and oxidative stress, and it may also help regulate blood sugar. Basically, wheatgrass has got it going on, and you'd be wise to get your hands on it.

Wheatgrass is surprisingly easy to come by: many health stores carry it, and you can even get a shot at Jamba Juice and Whole Foods coffee and smoothie bars. There are home delivery services, and it's also easy (and cheap) to grow.

Centrifugal juicers can't handle wheatgrass, so don't bother. You'll create mess and mayhem. In order to juice wheatgrass, you'll need a masticating or twin gear juicer or a hand-crank model.

Wheatgrass juicers work by slowly squeezing juice out of the tough wheatgrass fibers—similar to wringing out your wet clothes after running through the sprinkler.

Popular choices for hand-crank juicers: Lexen Healthy Juicer, Z-Star Manual Juicer, Chef's Star Manual Hand Crank, Handy Pantry HJ Hurricane. For electric versions, see my recommendations for masticating and twin gear juicers.

Wheatgrass may not taste like sunshine, but it will make you glow from the inside out. By the way, taking a sip of orange, pineapple, or apple juice as a chaser will help to balance out wheatgrass's eau de earthiness.

process of making a juice tends to take a bit longer than centrifugal. The prep involves cutting the produce into smaller sizes because their mouths are typically narrow. Feeding the juicer takes time because the gears turn slowly. And finally, the cleanup can include a few extra steps because there are often more parts to rinse and scrub. In addition, sometimes pulp can slip through. No biggie. You can either strain it or just enjoy the extra fiber.

These juicers are also more expensive. All that said, they're still the go-to choice for health gurus and advocates.

Consider all of these factors when you're thinking about the juicer you want; there's no point having a fancy machine if the time you need to spend cleaning it outweighs your juice craving in the first place!

Popular choices for twin gear juicers: Super Angel 5500, Samson Green Power, Green Star Elite Juice Extractor.

ENZYMES

Enzymes are your body's workforce. They're the busy builders and demolition teams that constantly tear down and reconstruct the body. Millions of enzymes are working in your body right now to support everything from digesting your green juice to healing your paper cut.

Digestive enzymes help break down food, while metabolic enzymes run the rest of the show by orchestrating the biochemical reactions that fuel every cell in your body. High temperatures destroy enzymes, so some experts believe that maximizing your intake of raw foods and fresh juices can help to replenish your body's reserve. Plus, the enzymes in certain fruits—pineapple, for instance—have a beneficial impact on digestion.

As you select a juicer, keep in mind that masticating and twin gear models will keep more enzymes intact—and allow them to last longer—than centrifugal machines.

Norwalk Hydraulic Press

Last but not least: the slowest, most effective badass on the scene. If you've won the lottery, robbed a bank, or inherited the family jewels from your aunt Trudy, check out the Norwalk juicer—which costs around $2500. This machine literally presses (as in uses a hydraulic press) the juice out of fruits and veggies, including tough-to-juice grasses like wheatgrass. This powerful juicer provides 50 to 100 percent more juice than other machines, and the juice itself will stay very fresh for up to three days.

Because Norwalk machines are so expensive, they're used mostly at healing centers or for commercial purposes—including the cold-pressed juices you may have come across in juice bars. You can't walk into the local Target and buy one. Generally, you have to procure them online or from a juice bar that sells them. But, hey, a gal can dream!

Before You Select a Juicer . . .

. . . ask yourself the following questions:

What's my budget?

How much prep time am I willing to invest in my daily juicing?

How much cleanup will I be willing to do on a daily basis?

What's more important: the shelf life of my juice or the time/effort it takes to prepare it?

How much space do I have?

Will I be juicing wheatgrass?

You can't go wrong with any of the juicers I've recommended. Keep that bad boy visible so you don't forget it exists. Clean it as soon as you're done using it so it's always ready to whip up a juice. If for whatever reason you can't clean it right away, soak the parts in warm water till you're ready. This will keep them from getting crusty (and stinky) and doubling the time it takes to clean.

Plus, if you have a pushy partner or husband like I do, cleaning the juicer right away will ensure a heavenly, lecture-free morning. For centrifugal juicers that have a catch basket, you can line it with a biodegradable bag for no-fuss-or-muss cleaning. Many juicers come with a scrub brush; this is essential for cleaning the basket or the nooks and crannies of the gears. If your juicer doesn't come with a brush, grab one the next time you're at the grocery store. It's the only way you'll get that sucker clean.

Look at your juicer purchase as a fresh start. You've taken your first step toward a glowing new you! Celebrate by drinking your first green juice in a champagne glass and toast to your health.

Crafting the Perfect Juice Combo

This book will give you plenty of inspiration for kick-ass, creative concoctions. But if you're a curious kitchen-lover like me, you'll want to build your own works of art. Here's some general guidance to help you choose the ingredients that tend to work best for crafting the perfect elixir. And don't fret—you can't make a mistake, and we'll talk all about specific ingredients in Chapter 4.

PICK YOUR BASE. The best bases are watery vegetables, which produce a lot of volume. My faves? Super-alkaline cucumber, electrolyte-rich celery, and even power-house broccoli stems work really well. Beets and carrots are also good, but a little goes a long way, as these root veggies contain more sugar. Of course, you don't have to pick just one base ingredient; a mixture of any of these veggies will work. The more, the merrier. Occasionally, I'll use fruit as a base for a light and fun alternative, but for the most part, watery veggies are my go-to for everyday juicing.

Cuisinart, Omega, Waring, and KitchenAid all make solid machines with prices ranging from $100 to $400.

Last but not least, there are the personal blenders, of which the Magic Bullet and Nutribullet are currently the most popular. Personal blenders are small (typically for making 1 to 2 servings at a time), affordable, and easy to use. These units are great for people who are challenged for counter space or who want to make smoothies on the road. They're a snap to clean and usually come with multiple pitcher sizes and blades. The Bullets have diehard fans, and if you enjoy binge-watching infomercials as much as I do, you've probably seen these superstars on the tube. Check them out!

Another option is the Vitamix S30. This little cutie is a dynamo of power. It comes with two small containers and a mini tamper (to make life easier and smoothies blend faster). I love using it to whip up smaller smoothie batches or to make sauces and dressings. It's easier than hauling out the big boys. Don't expect to pack it in your suitcase, though. It may be small, but it's still pretty heavy.

Before buying any blender, do your homework—research, read consumer reviews, and comparison-shop for the best deal. With a little effort, you'll find a righteous beast that serves you well.

Before You Select a Blender . . .

. . . ask yourself the following questions:

What's my budget?

How powerful does my blender need to be?

How much space do I have?

How many people am I blending for?

If you're into baubles and bonuses, many of these blenders come with accessories. Me, I'm simple. I look for a workhorse motor, good blades, and a warranty. As you rely on your blender for a variety of culinary creations, don't be surprised if stuff breaks or wears out over time. For your basic needs, a lower price-point blender can certainly do the trick. But as I mentioned before, when finances allow, you'll definitely want to upgrade. Another benefit of high-speed blenders is that they're better at pulverizing produce and extracting more nutrients from the fiber/pulp. They're also good at blending trickier ingredients like nuts and the aforementioned dates. FYI—soaking your nuts (I always laugh when I type that) and dates definitely makes them easier to blend.

If you have a blender with multiple speeds, give it some foreplay by starting on low and working your way up. You both will have a better experience. Above all, make sure the lid is secure. Jackson Pollock smoothie art on your walls and windows ain't cute. Another great tip is to invest in some good spatulas in various widths. These

FREEZING FRUIT

I love using frozen fruit in my smoothies. It creates thicker blends—the kind you can eat with a spoon—and makes your smoothies super cool and refreshing. Here are some of my favorite frozen fruits to use as smoothie bases:

BANANAS: I always have a bag of frozen 'naners sitting in my freezer; I peel, chop, and freeze them as soon as they're turning brown. Once again, don't forget to peel your bananas *before* freezing; the skins are almost impossible to get off once they're frozen!

MELON: Cantaloupe, honeydew, and watermelon all freeze well and add frosty texture to smoothies. I cut them into chunks, bag 'em up, and toss in the freezer.

MANGO: Bananas may be the most popular smoothie base, but for those of you who don't like bananas or are allergic to them, frozen mangoes create a similarly creamy, sweet base for smoothies.

Freezing fruit for smoothies is actually a great way to preserve ripe fruits that are perched on the cusp of going bye-bye. If I see a carton of berries that's getting slightly mushy or a banana that's turning brown, off to the freezer it goes. You'll also find bags of fruit in the freezer section of your health-food store, but pound for pound, you'll be paying more for the convenience.

Super frosty smoothies mighty feel too chilly in the dead of winter, so I often use room temperature fruit in the colder months. If you do this, you'll probably need to add less liquid than you would with frozen fruit.

Balancing Your Fruits and Veggies

Before you use all of this beautiful new knowledge to create some stunning concoctions, I want to address the issue of balance. Many people get overwhelmed when trying to figure out how many fruits and veggies to use in their drinks. Some folks don't want too much sugar; others lean toward sweeter recipes because they don't want to be hit in the kisser by an all-kale punch. If you're hoping to keep your juices a little more balanced—and maximize your alkaline intake—then the following suggestions are for you. They'll help you to craft elixirs that feature healthy amounts of fruits and veggies.

The basic goal is to include more veggies and leafy greens than fruit in your daily routine. For instance, when I make my green lemonade (page 127), I use celery, cucumber, and leafy greens, along with one small-to-medium-sized apple—a perfect ratio of alkalizing green goodness to natural, fruity sweetness. You can extend this rule of thumb to nearly all of your green juices, and you'll quickly see that a smaller portion of fruit (or sweet, starchy veggies) goes a long way in making those powerful greens powerfully palatable.

Do you always have to use this formula? Nope, this isn't an exact science. That's why you'll find recipes in this book that don't always hold tightly to that rule. The point is to add more veggies than fruit to your juice on a regular basis. Sometimes I crave a fruity drink (like my Green & Gold, page 165, or my Pretty in Pink juice, page 167). These sweeter blends are a great way to celebrate the natural sweetness and beauty of fresh fruit. But if you want to maximize the healing powers of your juices, then it's best to keep that ratio in mind most of the time.

It can be harder to stick to this ratio of more veggies to fruit when making smoothies, but try to work vegetables into your blended beverages whenever possible. Add a heaping amount of spinach, kale, or other

GREEN POWDERS

You may have seen commercial green powders on the market. These are usually a blend of chlorophyll, wheatgrass powder, barley grass powder, and other good green stuff. It may be tempting to use these powders in place of your own green drinks, but I recommend sticking to real produce. It's fresher and better for you than anything you can buy in a pouch.

That said, green powders are useful when you're on the go, traveling, or stuck at the office all night. Mix them into water for a boost. Green powders are also handy if you're low on veggies. My favorite brands include Amazing Grass, Aloha, and Garden of Life Perfect Food Green.

NUT/SEED MILK ICE CUBES

Yes, you read that correctly—this next tip is wicked good. When I was a smoothie newbie, I often struggled with runny, watered-down blends. I loved adding ice to them for a cool, frosty texture, but as the ice melted, so did the flavor. (Boo!) The discovery of nut milk ice cubes transformed my world, and it can revolutionize your smoothie-making process, too.

Simply set aside an ice-cube tray or two for nut milk cubes and fill them with nut, seed, or coconut milk. Put them in the freezer, and ta-da! They'll freeze, just like regular ice cubes, resulting in the perfect blending secret weapon.

Nut milk or coconut milk ice cubes will melt as you blend them, but instead of adding water to your blend, they'll add creamy, cool, nut milk texture. Pretty magical, right?

leafy greens to your blender, or try adding cucumber. (It's magical when whipped up with banana, mango, and other tropical fruits.) Carrots or carrot juice, beets, herbs, and even broccoli make wonderful smoothie additions—I promise!

Bottom line: If focusing on fruit in your smoothies helps you to get the green stuff in, then don't worry too much about your vegetable-to-fruit ratio. But over time, see if you can get into the habit of adding more

greens. Your taste buds will adapt, and it won't be long before you're hankering to get your greens.

The Glycemic Index & Glycemic Load

As you shift your focus away from processed sweets and toward naturally sweet fruits, it's helpful to keep a little system called the glycemic index (GI) in mind. The glycemic index is a measure of how quickly and how high a particular carbohydrate raises your blood sugar level. It's based on a numerical ranking system that compares a particular food to pure glucose (which is given a rating of 100). The closer a food's glycemic index is to 100, the more likely it is that its carbohydrates will raise blood sugar levels.

Foods with a very high GI value are almost always refined carbs—grain products, like white flour, that have had most of the fiber and nutrition stripped away, or white sugars and syrups. Conversely, foods that are low on the GI scale tend to be complex carbohydrates (think whole grains, like oats, brown rice, quinoa, and millet, or starchy root vegetables). These foods contain carbohydrates, but they don't cause blood sugar spikes the way refined carbs do, because their naturally occurring fiber and protein help to slow the entrance of sugar into the blood. Blood sugar spikes lead to insulin spikes, because insulin is the hormone that signals our body to store any sugar we don't immediately need. Over time, repeated insulin spikes can lead to weight gain and metabolic syndrome and other diseases.

When it comes to fruits, here's what you should know: lower-GI fruits include lemons, Granny Smith apples, berries, pears, grapefruit, oranges, grapes, and kiwi. Some higher-GI fruits include watermelon, grapes, bananas, pineapple, and dates.

In recent years, our understanding of the glycemic index has been refined, and another measure called the glycemic load (GL) has entered the picture. While the glycemic index only measures how quickly a carbohydrate is digested and converted into glucose in the bloodstream, the glycemic load takes into account how much of the carbohydrate we actually consume in one sitting. As it turns out, many of the fruits that have a high GI ranking actually have a low GL ranking, in part because we don't consume many of their carbohydrates per serving. Watermelon, for instance, has a GI of 72, but a GL of only 4. This is because watermelon is mostly water, so one serving actually doesn't supply us with much of the carbohydrate in question. The same goes for carrots, which have a GI of 71 but a GL of only 6. It's also true for bananas, grapes, and a number of other fruits.

So it's important to understand that a high GI ranking isn't the entire story and doesn't automatically mean that a fruit or vegetable is "bad." The glycemic load is often a better real-world indicator of how foods affect us, and it will help you compare some of your favorite juice and smoothie ingredients for their impact on blood sugar.

You can check out GI and GL rankings for a number of common foods at www.health.harvard.edu/healthy-eating/glycemic_index_and_glycemic_load_for_100_foods. For even more comprehensive information on glycemic index and glycemic load, check out *The New Glucose Revolution* by Jennie C. Brand-Miller, Ph.D.; Thomas Wolever, M.D.; Kaye Foster-Powell; and Stephen Colagiuri, M.D. Those folks are thorough! You can also

HOW TO ADJUST THE SUGAR CONTENT OF A RECIPE

Suppose you're being especially mindful of your sugar intake, but you fall in love with a juice or a smoothie recipe that seems to be on the sweeter side. Don't worry: most recipes can be modified to decrease sugar while retaining their character and flavor.

Start by examining what the sources of sweetness in the recipe are (sweet fruits, root vegetables, etc.) and decreasing the quantity of these ingredients. For example, if a juice calls for two or three apples, try using one instead. Or use Granny Smith apples rather than a sweeter variety. The important thing is to replace the sweet ingredient with another, lower-sugar one so that your yield stays consistent. I love to use cucumber and celery to create volume and flavor in recipes with minimal sugar (and maximal nutrition!). One medium cucumber will yield about the same amount of juice as two apples or three large carrots.

In smoothies, you'll often see a lot of banana, pineapple, or mango. If you prefer, replace some or all of these fruits with lower sugar options, like kiwi, peaches, pears, grapes, or berries.

Some of the smoothie recipes in this book call for pitted dates as a sweetener. Dates are one of the most concentrated sources of sweetness that nature has to offer. (They're called "nature's candy" for a reason.) I love using them in place of conventional syrups or refined sugars because they deliver caramel-like sweetness along with fiber, potassium, and magnesium. Usually, when I include dates in recipes, I'll give you a range in suggested quantity, so you can adjust the amount to fit your taste. You can also eliminate dates altogether. You know your body best.

These same principles work in reverse. If a juice or smoothie seems to lack the sweetness you crave, feel free to add a little more fruit, sweeter root veggies, or another date (in the case of smoothies). It's best to add these ingredients slowly because once your beverage has been sweetened, it's harder to tone it down if you've gone too far.

Finally, remember that it's possible to create tons of flavor and character in recipes without relying exclusively on sweet ingredients. One of my favorite tricks for brightening the taste of my juices and smoothies is to use fresh herbs, lemon, lime, and ginger. Just because your juice or smoothie isn't sweet, doesn't mean it should be blah.

find plenty of charts and information online.

Nutrition is complicated business, and how we respond to different ingredients depends heavily on our individual constitutions as well as our overall diet and lifestyle habits. Use the GI/GL for guidance, but don't go too crazy with it. Just make an overall effort to remember which foods are a bit higher on the spectrum, and if you're working with a health challenge, use the system as a means of creating the boundaries you need.

3

PREPPING
YOUR
KITCHEN

Once you've mastered your produce shopping routine, dive into stocking your pantry. Bulk bins and shelves lined with superfoods will become a happy haven. (See page 85 for more details on my favorite superfood finds.)

When to Buy Organic

When talking produce, one of the most common questions I get is: How important is it to buy organic?

Easy: buy organic as much as possible. This allows you to maximize your nutrient intake, avoid common pesticides and toxins, and support farmers who are doing their best to choose healthier methods for the planet and for us. Organic fruits and vegetables taste better and have consistently been shown to contain higher amounts of vitamins and minerals than nonorganic produce.

The problem, of course, is that organics are generally more expensive and not universally available (although on both accounts things are changing for the better). If you've got the money and the access, go 100 percent organic. But if you're like most people, that may be difficult. The good news is you don't have to be perfect in order to eat safer and healthier. That's because when it comes to pesticides and other toxins, not all produce is created equal. Some absorb more of the bad stuff during conventional farming, while others absorb very little. If you buy organic for just the few worst offenders while allowing nonorganic for the least,

you'll be in good shape without breaking the bank. My friends at the Environmental Working Group created the incredibly helpful "Dirty Dozen" and "Clean Fifteen" lists. Think of these must-haves as your shopping road map: memorize them, print them out, download their app—whatever it takes for you to use them. Keep in mind that they get updated yearly, so you'll want to check back in for the most current recommendations.

If you can't shop organic, period, that's okay, too. The most important thing is that you juice and blend those fruits and veggies! If you're juicing nonorganic produce (like cucumbers, carrots, or apples), just be sure to peel them first and wash them thoroughly before running them through your juicer. For more tips on washing produce, check out page 66.

Tips for Saving Money

While we're on the topic of grocery shopping, let's talk budgeting. As you already know, all of the gorgeous, organic produce you plan to stock your kitchen with can add up. But it's definitely less expensive than doctors' bills, excessive medications for lifestyle-related ailments, missed days at work due to poopy health, and so on. It'll take a little extra time and effort, but if you'd like to make juices and smoothies less of a strain on your purse strings, try adopting a few of these helpful habits. (You'll also be

THE DIRTY DOZEN

1. APPLES
2. PEACHES
3. NECTARINES
4. STRAWBERRIES
5. GRAPES
6. CELERY
7. SPINACH
8. SWEET BELL PEPPERS
9. CUCUMBERS
10. CHERRY TOMATOES
11. SNAP PEAS (IMPORTED)
12. POTATOES
13. *RUNNER UP:* HOT PEPPERS
14. *RUNNER UP:* KALE / COLLARD GREENS

THE CLEAN FIFTEEN

1. AVOCADOS
2. SWEET CORN
3. PINEAPPLE
4. CABBAGE
5. SWEET PEAS (FROZEN)
6. ONIONS
7. ASPARAGUS
8. MANGOES
9. PAPAYAS
10. KIWI
11. EGGPLANT
12. GRAPEFRUIT
13. CANTALOUPE
14. CAULIFLOWER
15. SWEET POTATOES

doing Mama Earth a solid when you follow some of these suggestions.)

SUPPORT YOUR LOCAL FARMERS' MARKETS. Farmers' market produce isn't always cheap, but farmers will often offer specials on fruits and vegetables that are at the height of freshness. You may be able to get your haggle on at your local market, too—particularly at the end of the day when farmers don't want to pack up what didn't sell.

JOIN A CSA. Here's how it works: in the winter, you buy an advance share of the produce that a particular farmer or co-op plans to grow for the year ahead. When the crop starts coming, you swing by the farm (or a set pick-up location) and grab your share on a designated day. It's amazing how many bags of fresh greens you'll start to see in early spring—in fact, you may not be able to make it through all of your produce, in which case you can go halvsies with a friend.

A CSA share usually runs about $400 to $500 a year—sometimes less if you choose a smaller package. This sounds like a lot of money, but once you start collecting sexy sacks of fabulous produce each week, I guarantee you'll realize it's a huge bargain. Don't just take my word for it, though; crunch some numbers and see if it makes sense for you. CSAs are also a great way to discover new, exotic produce since you don't always have a choice of what's in the weekly haul.

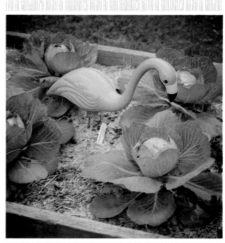

SHOP ONLINE. Another great way to save moolah is to shop online. Stores like Vitacost and Thrive Market have become virtual health hubs that offer great products at deep discounts. These companies also offer free or reasonable shipping prices. In the case of Thrive Market, there's an annual membership fee (similar to Costco) but with one big difference: when you buy a membership, Thrive gives one away to a low-income family! While these stores don't offer vegetables (yet) they're a great place to get bulk staples like superfoods and healthy sweeteners at near wholesale prices.

BUILD ON WHAT YOU HAVE. Examine your fridge and cupboards. What can you build on? What needs to be used up? If you have viable produce at home, then don't run out to purchase more just yet. Think about what fabulous recipes you can create with what you have.

MAKE PLANS. To avoid running low on fruits and vegetables, try to plan out your week of beverages before you shop. This will help you to resist sneaky impulse buys, shop more efficiently, and save money. Divide your grocery list into staples (the fruits and veggies you just can't live without), seasonal picks (stuff that's not necessarily a staple, but which you want to take advantage of by season, like apples in the fall or peaches in the summer), and splurges (superfood goodies). Think about what you can afford, and do some trimming from your list, if necessary. For a free downloadable meal plan, go to kriscarr.com. I love making helpful stuff for you!

WASTE NOT, WANT NOT. Leftover broccoli stems from last night's stir-fry? They're great in a juice! Got half an avocado from lunch? Let that be the base of your next creamy green smoothie. Fruit and veggie odds and ends are ideal for juicing and blending, so take advantage. One of the biggest causes of waste is buying too much, only to find a slimy mystery bag in the bottom of the crisper a week later. Live food has a short shelf life compared to those Twinkies, so plan wisely.

SAVVY SUBSTITUTIONS. If certain ingredients are weighing your budget down, look for more affordable alternatives. Raisins make a great substitute for pitted Medjool dates; sunflower seeds are cheaper than cashews, and they offer similar creaminess. Depending on the season, a particular type of green might be cheaper than the one that's called for in a recipe, so feel free to switch and swap. Check out the substitutions list on page 95 for help.

REVIEW THE DIRTY DOZEN AND THE CLEAN FIFTEEN. Check out the Environmental Working Group's lists (printed on page 60) to determine your priorities for organic purchases. Choose organic for produce on the Dirty Dozen list and conventional for the Clean Fifteen (or for most fruits and veggies that have thick skins).

LET YOUR GARDEN GROW. If you have space, start your own vegetable and herb garden. A two-dollar packet of mixed lettuce seeds will support your juicing habit for months. Even if you live in a major metropolis, you can still invest in growing your own greens and herbs. When I lived in Brooklyn, NY, I grew sprouts in my bathroom and herbs on my windowsill. Today I have a raised-bed garden in my backyard, and each year I learn more and more about how to grow our food (AKA not kill my plants).

There are many great books (and websites) on gardening. Here are a few of my favorite reads: *The Vegetable Gardener's Bible* by Edward C. Smith, *Grow Organic* by Doug Oster and Jessica Walliser, *Starter Vegetable Gardens* by Barbara Pleasant, and *You Grow Girl* by Gayla Trail (perfect for the urban gal or guy). Also, check out fourseasonfarm. com. Greening your thumb is easier than you think!

KEEP YOUR PRODUCE FRESH LONGER. Review the Ingredients Section (page 65) for proper storage tips that will extend the life of your fruits and veggies. When recommended, use those Debbie Meyer GreenBags I've been raving about like an excited lunatic.

BUY USED, OR BARTER. Buying a new juicer or blender may not be in your budget right now, but what about a used one?

The only caveat is that most of these used machines are not returnable and have no warranty—so ask for a test run before you buy. As I mentioned earlier, some companies do offer cheaper, reconditioned machines with warranties. Craigslist or eBay, not to mention your friends and family, might also have an affordable gently used model. Perhaps you can barter with those great boots that are too small for you. A purrrfect swap! Amazon, eBay, and Bed Bath & Beyond offer sales and competitive prices, so take time to do your homework.

SKIP THE FANCY ADD-ONS. Instead of buying every trendy superfood that can fit in a blender, try one at a time and slowly build up your arsenal. Go ahead and splurge once in a while, but if you're looking for somewhere to cut corners, skip the exotic stuff and focus your energy (and funds) on quality produce.

TIGHTEN YOUR BELT IN OTHER AREAS. Do you cruise Target looking for sparkly tanning lotions, huggable hangers, "deals," and "cheap" gadgets? I know you do, because I do. If you think about it, I'm sure you've got some frivolous spending habits you could lose. Redistribute your funds. Use them where they matter most. Remember that every single green drink you create is an investment in your quality of life—now and always.

4

SPOTLIGHT ON INGREDIENTS

Ahhh . . . the bountiful harvest. In this chapter, I'm going to open your purdy peepers to the ingredients that are the juicing and blending all-stars.

This info is divided into three sections: leafy greens, fruits and veggies, and superfood boosts. This definitive guide will show you how to pick, prep, and store your favorite foods. You'll also learn about the top nutrients and benefits of these plant gems—plus how to choose a substitute for those you'd rather avoid. Before we jump in, let's talk about how to clean these cuties.

Washing and Cleaning Produce

Before you put your gorgeous produce into the juicer or blender and down your glamorous gullet, it's important to be sure that you've washed off bacteria, debris, sand, and dirt. Most resources suggest that fresh produce should be washed under tap water for at least 30 seconds to remove dirt and microorganisms. (Rinsing is better than soaking, because sinks and soak containers can harbor little critters!) Use a scrub brush for hard surfaces like beets, carrots, and cucumbers. For leafies and other delicates, rinse and rub gently. Nonorganic produce should always be washed to help remove pesticide residues. Food scientists have found that using water is just as effective as standard fruit and vegetable washes.

Depending on your health needs and circumstances, there are a few other cleaning options you can use:

Flash Pasteurization: This is an aggressive but reliable means of making sure that produce ends up squeaky clean and bacteria-free—which may be important to those who are immunocompromised (for example, if you're going through a treatment such as chemotherapy). Bring a pot of water to boil, then dip your veggies in it for no more than 20 seconds. Fragile greens need only about 5 seconds. This procedure will kill most, if not all, the germs while keeping nutrients intact.

Hydrogen Peroxide Vegetable Soak: This option reliably removes bacteria and is another suitable method for those who may have weakened immune systems. However, it's very important that you follow precautions or serious injury can occur. Food-grade hydrogen peroxide is typically available in a 35 percent solution. This is a very strong concentration and can burn skin on contact. It must be diluted with water down to 3 percent before using to clean your food. Do an online search for help with proper dilution.

White Vinegar Vegetable Soak: You can also try white vinegar for cleaning your produce. Fill a large bowl with water and add about a half cup of vinegar. Let your veggies (or fruits) sit for about 20 minutes before rinsing and using.

Spotlight on Greens

Say hello to your new BFF, greens! These babies are nutrient-dense stunners. The more you embrace them, the happier and healthier your body will be.

Arugula

SELECTION: Choose arugula with long, firm, bright green leaves without holes, tears, or bright yellow edges.

STORAGE: Store in the vegetable drawer of the fridge for 2 to 3 days.

PREPARATION FOR USE: Wash thoroughly to remove dirt and grit.

TOP NUTRIENTS: carotenoids beta-carotene, lutein, and zeaxanthin, vitamin K, sulforaphane, chlorophyll

HEALTH BENEFITS: promotes healthy eyes and skin, fights cancer, boosts immunity, builds healthy bones, helps in blood clotting, detoxifies the body, builds and purifies blood, revitalizes cells, combats inflammation

Collards

SELECTION: Leaves should be firm and deep green with no signs of wilting or yellowing.

STORAGE: Unwashed greens can be stored in the fridge in a plastic bag with as much air removed as possible for 4 to 6 days.

PREPARATION FOR USE: Wash leaves individually, making sure to remove all dirt and grit. Bunch or roll up the leaves before running them through your juicer, taking care to follow them with a more watery fruit or vegetable (apples, cucumber, celery, carrot, pineapple, etc.). Most leaves are a suitable size for blending, but larger leaves can be sliced in half if necessary.

TOP NUTRIENTS: carotenoid beta-carotene, vitamin C, vitamin K, calcium, choline

HEALTH BENEFITS: promotes healthy eyes and skin, fights cancer, boosts immunity, acts as an antioxidant, builds healthy bones, helps in blood clotting, helps keep blood pressure down, boosts memory, may help lower cholesterol

Dandelion greens

SELECTION: Leaves should be flat, crisp, unwilted, and bright green without any yellowing.

STORAGE: Unwashed greens can be stored in a plastic bag in the low-moisture veggie drawer in the fridge for up to 5 days.

PREPARATION FOR USE: Wash thoroughly to remove all dirt and grit.

TOP NUTRIENTS: carotenoids lutein and zeaxanthin, vitamin C, vitamin K, calcium

HEALTH BENEFITS: promotes healthy eyes and skin, fights cancer, boosts immunity, combats inflammation, acts as an antioxidant, builds healthy bones, helps in blood clotting, helps keep blood pressure down, detoxifies the body

Kale

SELECTION: Leaves should be unwilted, small to medium in size for best tenderness, deep green in color with no yellowing or browning, and stems should be moist.

STORAGE: Store unwashed in a plastic bag in the fridge with as much air removed as possible to maintain freshness for up to 5 days. The longer kale sits in the fridge, the more bitter it will become.

PREPARATION FOR USE: Wash leaves individually to remove all dirt and grit. If your leaves are very large, you can juice them one by one. For most bunches of kale (any variety—curly, purple, or lacinato), you can juice three or four leaves at a time.

TOP NUTRIENTS: carotenoids beta-carotene and lutein, vitamin C, vitamin K, calcium, copper, isothiocyanates

HEALTH BENEFITS: promotes healthy eyes and skin, fights cancer, boosts immunity, acts as an antioxidant, builds healthy bones, helps keep blood pressure down, supports proper growth, aids in energy production, acts as an antimicrobial, detoxifies the body

Romaine

SELECTION: The head should be closely bunched and leaves should be crisp without any slimy or dark spots, or any browning or wilting.

STORAGE: Wash and dry leaves with a paper towel and then store in a plastic bag in the fridge for up to a week.

PREPARATION FOR USE: Separate leaves and submerge them in a bowl of water, moving them around to help remove dirt and grit, and then rinse them individually. Run the leaves through your juicer several at a time, or break them up before blending.

TOP NUTRIENTS: carotenoid beta-carotene, folic acid, vitamin K

HEALTH BENEFITS: promotes healthy eyes and skin, fights cancer, boosts immunity, combats inflammation, supports healthy cells and genetic material, builds healthy bones, helps in blood clotting

Spinach

SELECTION: Choose crisp, green bunches with no evidence of insect damage.

STORAGE: Wrap loosely in a damp paper towel and store in the fridge in a plastic bag for 3 to 5 days.

PREPARATION FOR USE: Submerge leaves in a bowl of water, moving them around to help remove dirt and grit. Rinse the leaves. For best results when juicing, bunch spinach up before running it through your juicer.

TOP NUTRIENTS: carotenoids beta-carotene, lutein, and zeaxanthin, folic acid, vitamin K, copper, iron, manganese

HEALTH BENEFITS: promotes healthy eyes and skin, fights cancer, boosts immunity, combats inflammation, supports healthy cells and genetic material, builds healthy bones, helps in blood clotting, supports proper growth, aids in energy production, improves oxygen transport throughout the body, promotes the healthy metabolism of fats and carbohydrates

Fruit and Vegetable All-Stars

Meet my favorite fruits and vegetables! They're bound to perk you up and add yum to your recipes.

Swiss chard

SELECTION: Leaves should be vivid green with no signs of wilting or browning. Stalks should be crisp and undamaged.

STORAGE: Store, unwashed, in an airtight plastic bag in the fridge for up to 5 days. Extra chard can be blanched and frozen for 1 month.

PREPARATION FOR USE: Separate chard leaves from the bunch and wash individually, taking care to rinse the stems well. (This is where dirt and grit can collect.) Bunch the leaves up before running them through your juicer, taking care to follow them with a more watery fruit or vegetable (apples, cucumber, celery, carrot, pineapple, etc.).

TOP NUTRIENTS: carotenoids beta-carotene, lutein, and zeaxanthin, vitamin C, vitamin K, copper, magnesium, quercetin, kaempferol

HEALTH BENEFITS: promotes healthy eyes and skin, fights cancer, boosts immunity, acts as an antioxidant, builds healthy bones, helps in blood clotting, supports proper growth, aids in energy production, increases muscle relaxation for improved blood flow, promotes heart health

Apples

SELECTION: Fruit should be firm, colorful, and not at all wrinkled or yielding to pressure. Brown spots are okay and rarely affect taste.

STORAGE: Store in perforated plastic bag in refrigerator for up to 4 months.

PREPARATION FOR USE: Wash and core apples, removing the seeds. For juicing, be sure to cut them into pieces that are small enough to fit through the juicer mouth (to help avoid juicing traffic jams). If your apples aren't organic, peel them.

TOP NUTRIENTS: vitamin C, anthocyanins (in red-skinned apples)

HEALTH BENEFITS: acts as an antioxidant, combats inflammation, fights cancer, prevents heart disease

Avocados

SELECTION: Ripe avocados are slightly soft when pressed, and dark in color; firm

avocados will ripen in 3 to 5 days. Avoid ones with sunken spots, cracks, or dull color.

STORAGE: Use ripe avocados immediately or store them in the fridge for up to 1 week. Placing unripe avocados in a paper bag may speed up ripening by 1 day, or they can be placed in the fridge to slow down the ripening process. Leftover avocados can be stored in the fridge with the pit, sprinkled with lemon juice, and wrapped in plastic wrap to avoid browning.

PREPARATION FOR USE: Cut your avocado in half lengthwise and use a small spoon to scoop out the pit. Scoop out flesh with a larger spoon before adding it to smoothies.

TOP NUTRIENTS: vitamin B5 (pantothenic acid), folic acid, vitamin E, vitamin K, potassium

HEALTH BENEFITS: detoxifies the liver, supports healthy cells and genetic material, acts as an antioxidant, builds healthy bones, helps in blood clotting, helps keep blood pressure down

USING AVOCADO

Avocado (AKA nature's butter) is a magical smoothie muse; more than any other ingredient, it'll add a creamy, almost fluffy texture to your blends. Be careful not to add too much, though, or your blend will resemble a pudding more than a smoothie (which, on second thought, sounds divine). I find that half of a small Hass avocado is a perfect amount. Avocado pairs particularly well with tropical fruits, berries, and greens.

STORAGE: Ripen bananas at room temp. Peel and freeze ripe or overripe (all brown) bananas in a plastic bag for smoothies for up to 6 months.

PREPARATION FOR USE: Peel and freeze before blending if possible.

TOP NUTRIENTS: vitamin B6, vitamin C, potassium, manganese

HEALTH BENEFITS: maintains sodium-potassium balance in your body, promotes red blood cell production, acts as an antioxidant, helps keep blood pressure down, promotes the healthy metabolism of fats and carbohydrates

Bananas

SELECTION: Choose bananas that are firm, vibrant yellow, and without bruises. They taste the sweetest when they have small brown spots.

Basil

SELECTION: Choose organic (nonirradiated), fresh leaves that are vibrant and deep green without dark spots.

STORAGE: Store wrapped in a damp paper towel for up to 5 days in the fridge. It can be chopped and frozen in an airtight container and kept for up to 6 months.

PREPARATION FOR USE: Submerge the basil—stems and leaves both—in a bowl of water and swish it around to release all dirt. Shake it dry before running it through your juicer or adding it to smoothies. If your herbs seem spiffy, then it's fine to simply rinse them well before using.

TOP NUTRIENTS: vitamin K, manganese, flavonoids, volatile oils

HEALTH BENEFITS: builds healthy bones, helps in blood clotting, promotes the healthy metabolism of fats and carbohydrates, combats inflammation

Beets

SELECTION: Choose small- or medium-sized beets with smooth skin and deep color. Avoid beets that have spots or bruises, or are shriveled or flabby.

STORAGE: Store in a plastic bag in the fridge for up to 3 weeks.

PREPARATION FOR USE: Trim the tough ends off, then wash the beets and cut them into pieces that will fit into the mouth of your juicer.

TOP NUTRIENTS: folic acid, manganese, potassium, betalains

HEALTH BENEFITS: supports healthy cells and genetic material, promotes the healthy metabolism of fats and carbohydrates, helps keep blood pressure down, acts as a strong antioxidant

Bell peppers

SELECTION: Choose peppers that are heavy and have brightly colored, tight skin. Stems should be green and fresh looking. Avoid peppers with blemishes, spots, or wrinkles.

STORAGE: Store in a plastic bag in the fridge for up to 5 days.

PREPARATION FOR USE: Remove the stem of the pepper by cutting around it with a paring knife and gingerly pulling it out. This will remove most of the seeds. Wash and quarter the pepper before juicing or blending.

TOP NUTRIENTS: carotenoids alpha-carotene, beta-carotene, cryptoxanthin, lutein, and zeaxanthin, vitamin C, vitamin B6, flavonoids

HEALTH BENEFITS: promotes healthy eyes and skin, fights cancer, boosts immunity, acts as an antioxidant, maintains sodium-potassium balance in the body, promotes red blood cell production, combats inflammation

Blackberries

SELECTION: Choose berries that are shiny and very dark in color, not bruised or leaking.

STORAGE: Store unwashed in the fridge for 3 to 5 days and wash right before eating. Freeze extras in a plastic bag for up to 1 month.

PREPARATION FOR USE: Wash well before freezing, blending, or juicing.

PREPARATION FOR USE: Cut your melon into quarters and use a paring knife to remove skin. Be sure to scoop out the seeds.

TOP NUTRIENTS: vitamin C, potassium

HEALTH BENEFITS: acts as an antioxidant, helps keep blood pressure down

Jalapeño

SELECTION: Peppers should be brilliant in color with firm, glossy skin. Avoid those that are wrinkled or have soft spots.

STORAGE: Wrap in paper towels or in a paper bag and store in the fridge for up to 1 week.

PREPARATION FOR USE: Wash pepper, cut a desired piece, and use. Jalapeños are very (holy hotness) spicy, so be sure not to touch sensitive skin or rub eyes after you've handled them.

TOP NUTRIENT: vitamin C

HEALTH BENEFITS: acts as an antioxidant

Kiwifruit

SELECTION: Choose kiwifruit that is plump, unwrinkled, and unblemished. It is ripe when it yields slightly to pressure.

STORAGE: Fruit can be ripened at room temp in a paper bag with an apple or banana to speed up the process. Once ripe, store it in a sealed container in the refrigerator for up to 2 weeks.

PREPARATION FOR USE: Peel before juicing or blending.

TOP NUTRIENTS: vitamin C, vitamin K, potassium

HEALTH BENEFITS: acts as an antioxidant, builds healthy bones, helps in blood clotting, helps keep blood pressure down

Lemons

SELECTION: Choose fruit that is deep yellow, shiny, and heavy for its size. Avoid fruit that is wrinkled or dull in color.

STORAGE: Store at room temperature out of sunlight for up to 1 week and in the vegetable crisper of the fridge for up to 1 month.

PREPARATION FOR USE: Peel lemons and cut them to fit into your juicer. It's fine to leave the pith on. If using lemon juice in smoothies, squeeze and measure fresh juice and add it to your smoothie blend.

TOP NUTRIENTS: vitamin C, limonoids

HEALTH BENEFITS: acts as an antioxidant, fights cancer of the mouth, skin, lung, breast, stomach, and colon

PEELING CITRUS

There are many ways to peel citrus fruits (including lemons, limes, grapefruits, and oranges) for juices and smoothies. If you have a method that works for you, then it's fine to keep using it. I personally like to use a paring knife to slice off the ends of the citrus fruit. I then set the citrus fruit down on one of its two peeled ends, and I use my knife to cut the skin off in vertical strips, moving from the top of the fruit to the bottom.

It's not necessary to seed lemons, limes, oranges, or grapefruit for fresh juices. For smoothies, you'll need to remove seeds if you're using a conventional blender. If you're using a high-speed blender, it's okay to throw the fruit in, seeds and all!

Final note: though bitter to taste, the pith of an orange contains as much vitamin C as the fruit itself, so it's fine if some of it remains on the fruit before juicing or blending.

Limes

SELECTION: Choose plump limes that are heavy for their size with a deep green, glossy peel. Avoid ones that have a lot of brown on the peel, as they may have a moldy taste.

STORAGE: Store at room temperature out of sunlight for up to 1 week and in the vegetable crisper of the fridge for up to 1 month.

PREPARATION FOR USE: Peel limes and cut them to fit into your juicer. It's fine to leave the pith on. If using lime juice in smoothies, squeeze and measure fresh juice and add it to your smoothie blend.

TOP NUTRIENTS: vitamin C, limonoids

HEALTH BENEFITS: acts as an antioxidant, fights cancer of the mouth, skin, lung, breast, stomach, and colon

Pineapple

SELECTION: Pineapple should be heavy for its size and free of soft spots or dark "eyes," and have a pleasant aroma. Pineapple stops ripening as soon as it is picked, but it will get softer and juicier after a few days at room temperature.

STORAGE: Store uncut pineapple in a plastic bag in the refrigerator for up to 5 days. Store cut pineapple in some of its own juice in a sealed container for up to 3 days.

PREPARATION FOR USE: Cut off the top of the fruit and slice the pineapple into quarters. Cut out the woody core of the fruit and then use a paring knife to remove the skin.

TOP NUTRIENTS: vitamin C, manganese, bromelain

HEALTH BENEFITS: acts as an antioxidant, promotes the healthy metabolism of fats and carbohydrates, combats inflammation, slows the growth of tumor cells

Raspberries

SELECTION: Choose plump, tender berries that are uniform in color. Avoid leaking or moldy berries.

STORAGE: Store in the fridge in a non-airtight shallow container for 3 to 5 days and wash only right before eating. Freeze extras in a plastic bag for up to 1 month.

PREPARATION FOR USE: Wash well before freezing, blending, or juicing.

TOP NUTRIENTS: vitamin C, manganese, anthocyanins, ellagic acid, hydroxycinnamic acids, resveratrol

HEALTH BENEFITS: acts as an antioxidant, promotes the healthy metabolism of fats and carbohydrates, combats inflammation, acts as an antimicrobial, may cause cancer cell death, prevents heart disease

Strawberries

SELECTION: Choose berries that have a shiny, deep red color and attached green caps. Avoid those that are shriveled or moldy. Plan to eat strawberries within 3 days.

STORAGE: Remove soft or moldy strawberries from the group before storing the rest in an airtight container in the fridge. They should remain fresh for up to 3 days. Only wash right before eating.

PREPARATION FOR USE: Wash well before freezing, blending, or juicing.

TOP NUTRIENTS: vitamin C, manganese, anthocyanins, ellagic acid, hydroxycinnamic acids, resveratrol

HEALTH BENEFITS: acts as an antioxidant, promotes the healthy metabolism of fats and carbohydrates, combats inflammation, acts as an antimicrobial, may cause cancer cell death, prevents heart disease

Tarragon

SELECTION: Choose fresh tarragon that has bright green leaves that are not wilted, limp, or have dry brown or yellow areas.

STORAGE: Store in a sealed bag in the refrigerator crisper away from tomatoes, bananas, and peppers for up to 5 days.

PREPARATION FOR USE: Tarragon can be juiced or blended whole—stems and leaves. Most fresh herbs do contain some grit, so I recommend submerging them in a bowl of water and swishing them around to release the dirt. Shake them dry before using them. If your herbs seem spiffy, it's fine to simply rinse them well before using.

TOP NUTRIENT: eugenol

HEALTH BENEFITS: stimulates the appetite, acts as an antioxidant

Watermelon

SELECTION: Choose an uncut watermelon that is firm, shiny but slightly dulled on top, and heavy for its size (water content increases with ripening). The ground spot (where the melon was in contact with the soil) on a fully ripened watermelon will be creamy yellow, not light green or white. Cut watermelon should be deep pink in color.

STORAGE: Whole melons are ideally stored in a basement area where the temperature is cooler than room temp and warmer than the fridge (50 to 60 degrees Fahrenheit). Whole melons shouldn't be stored near ethylene-producing fruits like passion fruit, peaches, pears, apples, or papaya, as they may ripen too quickly. Once cut, store in an airtight container in the fridge for up to 3 days.

PREPARATION FOR USE: Cut watermelon into large wedges. Use a sharp knife to remove the rind and seeds, and cut watermelon pieces into large chunks.

TOP NUTRIENTS: lycopene, vitamin C

HEALTH BENEFITS: helps prevent prostate cancer, acts as an antioxidant

Superfood Boosts

"Superfood" is a big buzzword these days, and it can be hard to figure out what the term really means. Think of it this way: a superfood is any ingredient that happens to be incredibly rich in micronutrients (vitamins, minerals, and phytochemicals). As you'll see, many nuts and seeds (including coconut and pumpkin seeds) qualify as superfoods, as do a bunch of commonly used spices, like cinnamon.

There are a couple of specialty ingredients—many indigenous to South and Central America—that are labeled as superfoods because their nutrient profiles are so incredibly unique. These include maca, a libido-boosting tuber that's usually sold in powder form, and acai, an antioxidant-rich, deep purple berry that's native to Trinidad and northern regions of South America. These ingredients aren't essential for a healthy lifestyle, but they can be fun to experiment with, and while they're sometimes on the pricier side, fortunately, a little goes a long way.

Acai

SELECTION: Choose frozen acai puree (such as in a smoothie pack) that is unsweetened, organic, non-GMO, and free of preservatives or colorings.

STORAGE: Store in the freezer as long as package indicates (sometimes up to 5 years). Once thawed, store puree in the fridge and use within 2 days.

PREPARATION FOR USE: Acai is typically sold in frozen packs that can be added to smoothies. You can use half a pack or a whole pack at a time, depending on the recipe in question. Just be sure to purchase an unsweetened variety, per the above, as the sweetened acai packs can be very high in sugar.

TOP NUTRIENTS: vitamin C, calcium, anthocyanins, beta-sitosterol, essential fatty acids

HEALTH BENEFITS: acts as an antioxidant, combats inflammation, fights cancer, promotes heart health, lowers LDL (bad) cholesterol and increases HDL (good) cholesterol

Almonds

SELECTION: Choose raw almonds that are uniform in color, and not shriveled or limp. If buying in bulk, be sure inventory is turned over frequently. They should smell sweet and nutty, not sharp and bitter (those are rancid).

STORAGE: Store in an airtight container in a cool, dry place away from sunlight. Almonds stored in an airtight container in the fridge will last for several months.

PREPARATION FOR USE: Raw almonds should be soaked for 8 hours (or overnight) and rinsed before blending into smoothies or nut milks. See my tips on page 275 for more.

TOP NUTRIENTS: vitamin E, biotin, copper, manganese

HEALTH BENEFITS: acts as an antioxidant, strengthens hair, nails, and skin, may help lower cholesterol and improve blood sugar control, supports proper growth, aids in energy production, promotes the healthy metabolism of fats and carbohydrates

Aloe vera

SELECTION: Choose bottled juice that is organic, unflavored, in a BPA-free bottle, and free of sugar and preservatives. (I recommend the Lily of the Desert, Fruit of the Earth, or Nature's Way brands.)

STORAGE: Store according to bottle instructions. Bottled aloe vera juice can typically be stored in a cool, dark place for quite some time. Once opened, juice should be refrigerated and will typically last up to 2 months.

PREPARATION FOR USE: Simply measure liquid aloe vera from the bottle before adding to juices or smoothies.

TOP NUTRIENTS: lignins, saponins, essential fatty acids

HEALTH BENEFITS: reduces the risk of cancer and heart disease, enhances nutrient absorption, fights cancer, detoxifies the body, aids in digestion

Brazil nuts

SELECTION: Choose raw Brazil nuts that are whole, brown, heavy, and not shriveled or damaged. If buying in bulk, be sure inventory is turned over frequently. They should smell sweet and nutty, not sharp and bitter (those are rancid).

STORAGE: Store Brazil nuts in an airtight container a cool, dry place away from sunlight. Storing them in the fridge will increase their shelf life and help prevent them from going rancid.

PREPARATION FOR USE: Brazil nuts should be soaked for 4 hours and rinsed prior to blending in smoothies or nut milk (see my tips on page 275 for more). The nuts have a relatively soft, "buttery" texture, so if you have a high-speed blender, you can skip the soaking step if you forget.

TOP NUTRIENTS: copper, magnesium, phosphorus, selenium, essential fatty acids

HEALTH BENEFITS: supports proper growth, aids in energy production, increases muscle relaxation for improved blood flow, supports healthy bone formation, digestion, and hormone balance, acts as an antioxidant, promotes heart health, lowers LDL (bad) cholesterol, and increases HDL (good) cholesterol

Cacao / Cacao nibs

SELECTION: Choose organic.

STORAGE: Store nibs in an airtight container or bag with excess air squeezed out. Store at room temp or below in a dark area without sunlight exposure or moisture.

PREPARATION FOR USE: Measure your quantity of cacao nibs before blending and add the nibs directly to your blender. Cacao nibs take a few moments to blend completely. Cacao powder, on the other hand, will blend quickly and easily. It's more potent in taste than regular cocoa powder, so remember that a little will go a long way.

TOP NUTRIENTS: iron, catechins, anthocyanins

HEALTH BENEFITS: improves oxygen transport throughout the body, acts as an antioxidant, combats inflammation, acts as an antimicrobial, fights cancer, prevents heart disease

Cashews

SELECTION: Choose raw cashews with a sweet, nutty flavor.

STORAGE: Store in an airtight container in the fridge for up to 6 months or in the freezer for up to 1 year.

PREPARATION FOR USE: Soak cashews for between 2 and 4 hours and rinse before blending into nut milks or smoothies (see my tips on page 275 for more).

TOP NUTRIENTS: copper, magnesium, manganese, phosphorus, zinc

HEALTH BENEFITS: supports proper growth, aids in energy production, increases muscle relaxation for improved blood flow, promotes the healthy metabolism of fats and carbohydrates, supports healthy bone formation, digestion, and hormone balance, aids in healthy enzyme activity, boosts immunity

Cayenne

SELECTION: Choose organic powder.

STORAGE: Store in a tightly sealed glass jar out of sunlight for up to 6 months.

PREPARATION FOR USE: Add a small quantity of cayenne powder to smoothies or juices. Cayenne is very hot, so be mindful.

TOP NUTRIENTS: carotenoid beta-carotene, capsaicin

HEALTH BENEFITS: promotes healthy eyes and skin, fights cancer, boosts immunity, reduces pain, promotes heart health, acts as a nasal decongestant

Chia seeds

SELECTION: Choose organic chia seeds that don't stick together, or organic chia powder.

STORAGE: Store in an airtight container or bag at room temp for up to 1 year. Ground chia seeds can be stored in an airtight container in the fridge for up to 1 month.

PREPARATION FOR USE: Chia seeds can be added directly to a high-speed blender. If you're using a regular blender, try grinding your chia seeds in a coffee grinder, spice mill, or food processor prior to adding it to smoothies (you can use a 1:1 ratio for replacing whole chia with ground chia).

TOP NUTRIENTS: calcium, iron, protein, essential fatty acids

HEALTH BENEFITS: builds healthy bones, helps keep blood pressure down, improves oxygen transport throughout the body, promotes heart health, lowers LDL (bad) cholesterol, and increases HDL (good) cholesterol

Cinnamon

SELECTION: Sticks or powder should have a sweet smell indicating that it's fresh.

STORAGE: Store in a tightly sealed glass container in a cool, dark, dry place. Powder will last up to 6 months, sticks will last up to 1 year.

PREPARATION FOR USE: If you're using cinnamon sticks, grate the desired amount of cinnamon powder prior to adding it to a regular blender (you can also use a spice mill). If you have a high-speed blender, you can add pieces of cinnamon stick directly to the blender, though it may be easier to use ground cinnamon for measurement purposes.

TOP NUTRIENTS: manganese, cinnamic acid

The superfoods in this list don't simply have to be used when you're juicing or blending. Explore different nut milks and use them as a vehicle for your superfood ingredients. In the winter, I love to gently warm up a cup of almond or macadamia nut milk over the stove and add some spices (turmeric, ginger, cardamom) or superfoods (like maca, cacao, or matcha green tea). It's cozy and healthy!

production, improves oxygen transport throughout the body, protects against chemical carcinogens

Macadamia nuts

SELECTION: Choose shelled nuts (raw if available) that are firm and shiny or oily.

STORAGE: Store shelled nuts in an airtight container in the fridge for 6 to 12 months.

PREPARATION FOR USE: Macadamia nuts should be soaked for between 2 and 4 hours and rinsed before blending into smoothies

or nut milks (see my tips on page 275 for more). The nuts have a relatively soft, "buttery" texture, so if you have a high-speed blender, you can skip the soaking step in a pinch.

TOP NUTRIENTS: vitamin B1, manganese, selenium

HEALTH BENEFITS: aids in the healthy breakdown of fats, protein, and carbohydrates, acts as an antioxidant

Matcha green tea powder

SELECTION: Choose organic matcha powder that is unsweetened and bright green in color.

STORAGE: Store in a dark, cool, dry place, or in the fridge or freezer, but sealed tightly and away from strong smells, as it will take on neighboring aromas.

PREPARATION FOR USE: Can be added directly in specified amounts to smoothies. The powder can also be stirred by the quarter or half teaspoon into hot water for tea.

TOP NUTRIENTS: vitamin A, epigallocatechin gallate (EGCG)

HEALTH BENEFITS: promotes healthy eyes and skin, fights cancer, boosts immunity

Pumpkin seeds

SELECTION: Choose organic, raw seeds. Avoid those with shriveling or any evidence of moisture.

STORAGE: Store in an airtight container in the fridge for up to 6 months.

PREPARATION FOR USE: Pumpkin seeds should be soaked for 8 hours (or overnight) and rinsed prior to blending into smoothies or seed milk. See my tips on page 275 for more.

TOP NUTRIENTS: copper, magnesium, manganese, phosphorus, zinc

HEALTH BENEFITS: supports proper growth, aids in energy production, increases muscle relaxation for improved blood flow, promotes the healthy metabolism of fats and carbohydrates, supports healthy bone formation, digestion, and hormone balance, aids in healthy enzyme activity, boosts immunity

Raisins

SELECTION: Choose plump, moist raisins with wrinkles, not hard or too dried out.

STORAGE: Store raisins in a cool, dry place away from moisture and humidity. Once opened, store in the refrigerator in an airtight container to lengthen life and freshness.

PREPARATION FOR USE: If you have a high-speed blender, you can blend raisins directly into smoothies. If you don't, you should soak raisins in warm water for at least 30 minutes and drain the soak water before blending them.

TOP NUTRIENTS: iron, potassium, anthocyanins, resveratrol

HEALTH BENEFITS: improves oxygen transport throughout the body, helps keep blood pressure down, combats inflammation, fights cancer, prevents heart disease

Beets: Carrots, radish, sweet potato

Blackberries: Blueberries, cherries, raspberries, strawberries

Blueberries: Blackberries, cherries, raspberries, strawberries

Broccoli: Cabbage

Cabbage: Broccoli

Cantaloupe: Honeydew, watermelon

Carrots: Sweet potato, beets, radish

Celery: Swiss chard, cucumber

Cherries: Blackberries, blueberries, raspberries, strawberries

Cilantro: Parsley

Coconut meat, young Thai: Avocado, banana

Coconut water: Water or watermelon juice

Collard greens: Kale, Swiss chard, spinach, dandelion greens, arugula

Cucumber: Celery, zucchini

Dandelion greens: Arugula, collard greens, kale, Swiss chard, spinach

Grapefruit: Orange

Grapes: Pear, apple, kiwi

Honeydew: Cantaloupe, watermelon

Kale: Arugula, collard greens, dandelion greens, Swiss chard, spinach

Kiwi: Apple, grapes, pear

Lemon: Lime

Lettuce (such as red leaf or Boston): Romaine

Lime: Lemon

Mango: Banana, peaches, nectarines, plums, pineapple

Maple syrup: Medjool dates

Medjool dates: Maple syrup

Mint: Basil

Nectarines: Peaches, plums, mango

Orange: Grapefruit, pineapple

Parsley: Cilantro

Peaches: Nectarines, plums, mango

Pear: Apple, kiwi, grapes

Pineapple: Orange, mango

Plums: Mango, nectarines, peaches

Radish: Sweet potato, beets, carrots

Raspberries: Blackberries, blueberries, cherries, strawberries

Romaine: Lettuce (such as red leaf or Boston)

Spinach: Arugula, collard greens, dandelion greens, kale, Swiss chard

Strawberries: Blackberries, blueberries, cherries, raspberries

Sweet potato: Beets, carrots, radish

Swiss chard: Celery, collard greens, kale, dandelion greens, spinach, arugula

Watercress: Arugula

Watermelon: Cantaloupe, honeydew

Zucchini: Cucumber

Nuts & Seeds

Almond butter: Peanut butter, soy nut butter, cashew butter, sunflower seed butter, coconut butter

Almonds: Walnuts, pecans, Brazil nuts, cashews, peanuts

Brazil nuts: Almonds, cashews, macadamia nuts

Cashews: Macadamia nuts, pine nuts, Brazil nuts

Coconut: Cashews, macadamia nuts, Brazil nuts, avocado

Hemp seeds: Sunflower seeds, pumpkin seeds, sesame seeds

Macadamia nuts: Cashews, Brazil nuts

Peanut butter: Almond butter, soy nut butter, cashew butter, sunflower seed butter, coconut butter

Peanuts: Almonds

Pecans: Walnuts, almonds

Pumpkin seeds: Sunflower seeds, hemp seeds

Sesame seeds: Sunflower seeds, pumpkin seeds, hemp seeds

Sunflower seeds: Pumpkin seeds, hemp seeds, walnuts

Walnuts: Almonds, pecans, sunflower seeds

If you're allergic to most tree nuts, but you're not allergic to coconuts, try using coconut butter or young Thai coconut meat in smoothies in place of nuts or nut butter.

If you're allergic to tree nuts but not to seeds, try using sunflower seeds, pumpkin seeds, sesame seeds, or sunflower seed butter, pumpkin seed butter, or tahini in their place.

If you're allergic to all tree nuts and seeds, try using avocado in place of nuts to create creaminess in smoothies, rice or oat milk in place of almond (or other nut) milk, and soy nut butter in place of nut butters.

Superfoods

Cacao powder: Carob powder

Goji berries: Raisins

Hemp seeds: Sunflower seeds, pumpkin seeds, sesame seeds

Matcha green tea powder: ¼ cup brewed and cooled green tea

5

STAYING
HOOKED

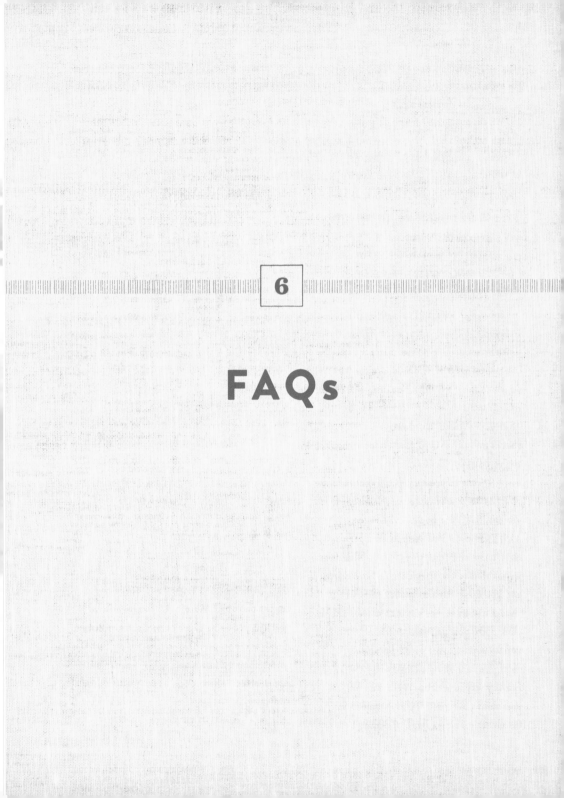

6

FAQs

their consumption of oxalates. Since raw greens contain more oxalates than cooked greens, a little caution about juicing and blending them in excess is reasonable for those at risk of stones.

It's important to remember that, for most of us, the benefits of incorporating more greens into our diets significantly outweigh the potential pitfalls. As with so many health questions, moderation is everything. Rotate your greens and, when you're not juicing or blending, cook them for variety. Juices and smoothies are kick-ass health boosters, but they're one piece of a well-rounded diet.

My juices and smoothies are: Just. Too. Green. Help!

Sister (and bro), this is a good problem to have. But if your juices bite you in the face with the taste of straight-up kale, then you may need to scale things back and add more watery veggies (like cucumber), plus a fruit. Zesty ingredients like lemon or ginger can mask the green while adding great flavor. Use our recipe collection as a guide.

How do I make my juice less pulpy?

So you thought the whole point of juicing was to remove fiber, but you keep finding bits of pulp in your juice (and your teeth). Wassup with that?

Certain types of juicers (like the Breville Fountain Crush Slow Juicer) are actually designed to keep some pulp in the juice. So, it's just a sign that the machine's doing its job! Other juicers may let a few bits of pulp through every now and then, which is pretty normal, but it could also mean that you're trying to pack in more produce than your juicer can handle. Ease up, hotshot. If you love making lots of juice at once, be sure to stop halfway through, open up the machine, and clear the pulp from the parts. Then you can reassemble and continue.

You can also try straining your juice through a sieve or nut milk bag before sipping. Voilà! Problem solved.

My juicer keeps jamming. What should I do?

Are you cutting your produce up into small enough pieces before juicing it? Even centrifugal juicers (which have nice, wide mouths) will jam if you stuff whole beets or apples in them. And remember that greens can give your juicer a hard time, so try to follow them up with something watery, like cucumber or apple (for more on this, see my tip on page 40). Most jams are caused when we're simply in too big of a rush. Take your time and don't force the plunger too hard. Let the machine do the work.

What do I do with leftovers if I make too much juice?

Well, the best solution is to make smaller quantities. But I personally love making extra. As I mentioned earlier, you can store fresh juice in a mason jar and keep it cold until you're ready to drink more. If you have a masticating juicer or a twin gear juicer, it can last up to a few days. The more sugar content in a recipe, the sooner it will go south. Pay attention to the color of the juice when you make it. It loses its vibrancy as a way of telling you, "Better drink me soon or I'm plant food." Yes, you can feed slightly expired juice to your grateful plants.

You can also freeze juice. This is a great tip if your time is limited and you'd prefer to make a big batch all at once. I recommend freezing juices either in BPA-free plastic water bottles or in mason jars. If you use mason jars, be sure to leave some space up at the top (about an inch or so) because your juices will expand as they freeze. Frozen juice will last for about 10 days, but be sure to freeze the juice immediately after you prepare it, to ensure freshness.

What should I do with my juice pulp?

So glad you asked! Don't despair, there's lots you can do with your pulp. Here are some of my favorite recycling ideas:

COMPOST. Juice pulp makes fabulous compost. How cool to think that we're using the scraps of our veggies to make our future veggie gardens grow! It's sorta like the "Circle of Life" song from *The Lion King,* but in your backyard.

CRACKERS. Juice pulp can be used to make delish, flour-free crackers. Check out the recipe on page 115 from my pal Gena Hamshaw, author of the blog and book *Choosing Raw.*

BURGERS. Want to infuse your homemade veggie burgers with even more fiber and texture? Check out the creative burger recipe on page 116, also from Gena Hamshaw.

If you do use your veggie juice pulp in a recipe, be sure to pick out tough, inedible seeds or other hard-to-digest bits before using, or else you'll end up with an impressive case of indigestion! Carrots, cucumber, leafy greens, and celery tend to make the best juice pulp.

How do I make my smoothies thicker?

Take a chill pill with the almond milk or coconut water. In other words, add less liquid. A cup and a half of nut milk is usually enough. To rescue a watery blend, pour it back in the blender and add half a 'nana, ¼ avocado, or another thickening ingredient. Frozen fruits create thicker blends than the same amount of fresh fruits.

How do I make my smoothies less thick?

This is an easy fix! If you're trying to pour your smoothie out of your blender and it won't budge, add a little more liquid. Start with a small amount—it doesn't take much to loosen it up. Add ¼ cup more nut milk, water, or coconut water at a time, and see if that does the trick.

juice pulp crackers

Makes about 24 to 30 crackers

2 heaping cups juice pulp (any veggies you like)

½ cup flax meal

3 tablespoons nama shoyu, tamari or (if you are gluten- and soy-free) coconut aminos

1 teaspoon coriander

½ teaspoon curry powder

Black pepper to taste (I'm generous with it)

¼ to ½ cup water

1. Blend all ingredients except for the water in a food processor. Add water to the food processor in a thin stream till the mix is easy to spread but not watery. (The amount of water you'll need will vary based on how watery the pulp is.)

2. *If you have a food dehydrator:* Turn the "dough" out onto a Teflex-lined dehydrator sheet and spread it evenly (it should be about ¼-inch thick, or just less than that). Score into cracker shapes with a knife or a pizza cutter. Dehydrate the crackers at 115 degrees Fahrenheit for about 4 hours. Flip the sheet by putting another Teflex sheet over it, flipping it over, and then peeling off your original sheet. Dehydrate for another 4 to 5 hours, or until crackers are nice and crunchy (again, this time may vary based on how watery your pulp was).

   If you don't have a food dehydrator: Preheat your oven to 325 degrees Fahrenheit. Spread the "dough" thinly (about ¼-inch thick, or just less) on a parchment-lined baking sheet and score into cracker shapes with a knife or a pizza cutter. Place the sheet in the oven. Bake for 30 to 40 minutes, or until the crackers are crispy and dry, flipping them halfway through baking.

3. Store the crackers in an airtight container in a cool, dry place.

juice pulp burgers

Makes 6 burgers

1 tablespoon + 2 teaspoons olive oil, divided

1 cup finely chopped onion

1 clove garlic, minced

½ cup pumpkin seeds, raw or toasted

½ teaspoon salt

Black pepper to taste

1 cup vegetable juice pulp (carrot, kale, spinach, cucumber, beet, or celery all work well)

1 cup cooked chickpeas (navy, aduki, and cannellini beans work, too)

¼ cup cooked quinoa

1 teaspoon flax meal

1 tablespoon lemon juice

2 teaspoons chopped fresh thyme (optional)

1 teaspoon paprika (optional)

⅓ cup water

1   Preheat your oven to 375 degrees Fahrenheit.

2   Heat 1 tablespoon of the olive oil in a skillet or sauté pan over medium heat. Add the onion and cook until the onion is tender and clear (5 to 7 minutes). Add the garlic and cook for another 30 seconds. Set aside.

3   Place the pumpkin seeds, salt, and pepper into the bowl of a food processor and process until they're coarsely ground. Add the juice pulp, chickpeas, quinoa, flax meal, lemon, thyme, and paprika, along with the water. Pulse the mixture continuously, until a sturdy dough has formed—sturdy enough to hold its shape, but moist enough that you can easily shape it into burgers (imagine a regular meatloaf or burger texture, even though this mixture is a little less uniform). If you need to add more water, do so by the tablespoon till the texture is right.

4   Shape the mixture into 6 uniform burger shapes. Place the burgers onto a parchment-lined baking sheet. Bake for 30 to 35 minutes, or until lightly browned, flipping them once halfway through. Leftover burgers will keep for 3 days in the fridge.

How do I stop my blender from getting stuck when I'm trying to make smoothies?

There's nothing worse than blender interruption! But this is an easy problem to fix. If you have a high-speed blender (like a Vitamix), then use the tamp attachment to push ingredients down as you blend. If you're working with a conventional blender, then stop once or twice mid-blending to mix the ingredients up with a spatula or wooden spoon. Just be sure that the blender is OFF before doing this; bark chips ain't tasty. If the problem persists, you may need to add some liquid (see previous FAQ).

I love smoothies, but I just can't handle the cold. Thoughts?

Are you suffering from brain freeze? Is there a blizzard outside your window, you're wearing three sweaters, and the mere thought of drinking something cold gives you hypothermia? My simple solution for this is to forgo frozen fruit and ice in recipes and use room temperature ingredients instead. It may also be helpful for you to start your day with more warming beverages and nourishing foods and enjoy your juices or smoothies later in the day after you've been more active. For a fabulous treat, try warming up your nut milks. Salud!

I'm constipated. What should I do?

FIRST QUESTION: Are you getting enough plant fiber in your diet? You may be juicing up a storm, but if you're skimping on fiber the rest of the time or you've been replacing a lot of your meals with juices, then your body may be crying out for more fiber to fuel its digestive engines. If so, incorporate more whole grains (including wheat-free grains like amaranth, quinoa, and teff), big salads, cooked vegetables, and legumes into your diet.

SECOND QUESTION: Has irregularity been a nagging part of your life for a while now? Then getting more beneficial bacteria into your diet may be helpful. You can explore fermented foods (sauerkraut, kombucha, kefir, tempeh, fermented veggies, miso), or you can consider a probiotic supplement. Some of these have dairy byproducts in them, but a few brands, including Rainbow Life's ProbioActive, Renew Life's Ultimate Flora, and Garden of Life's RAW probiotics, offer maximum probiotic power without any funky fillers or dairy. Avoid taking probiotic supplements along with any hot liquids, as the heat can kill off the good bugs.

Magnesium can also be a helpful supplement for those who are dealing with mild constipation. (And as an added bonus, it can help with stress relief!) I like the Natural Calm brand, which comes in a powder form. You can mix it into water and sip it before bed—a soothing ritual for your soul and your gut.

Finally, it's important to remember that,

even if you're flooding your diet with fresh juices and smoothies, the rest of what you eat still matters. Too many animal products, processed foods, and other nonalkaline munchies will take a toll. Many processed foods are very dehydrating, high in sodium, and tough to digest. The more you limit these foods and maximize your consumption of water, the better you'll be able to keep things moving and grooving.

You can also consider a colonic (AKA colon hydrotherapy). Don't be afraid. It's just a little hose and some water up your butt. You've done tougher things in your life—guaranteed. There are different types of colonic hydrotherapy. The most gentle, safe, and effective kind is called a gravity colonic. It allows warm water to gently enter your colon while also allowing you to release waste. The entire process is clean and odorless, facilitated by a certified therapist who may even tell you interesting stories to pass the time (and the poo). Anyway, colonics aren't needed on a regular basis, but if you're backed up, they can be super helpful. Just be sure to find a practitioner who is well respected, certified, and takes the time to make you feel comfortable and confident.

I'm making these drinks and I can't stop running to the bathroom. Help!

In all likelihood, one of two things is going on here. Either your body is responding to a flood of hydration from your juices, or it's dealing with an avalanche of fiber from your blends. In either case, diarrhea is your body's way of asking you to slow down (thank you very much). If you're consuming two or three juices or blends a day, try cutting back to one, and see how you feel. If you're blending up a ton of greens into your smoothies, try blending smaller amounts. Take it easy: juicing and blending is a lifelong love affair, not a race to the finish. If you see signs that tell you to slow down, heed them.

I'm feeling sluggish. Am I doing something wrong?

As we transition away from some of our favorite pick-me-ups throughout the day (Frappuccinos, Red Bulls, candy bars) it's completely normal to feel temporary dips in energy, a withdrawal from the chemical-induced stimulation that's been standing in for real energy. The good news is that the more good stuff you drink, the less you'll need or want your uppers. Give these juices and smoothies some time. They're not going to make your heart race (and pits sweat) the way a quad latte will. But if you make this a habit, they'll give your body the effortless and sustained energy it desires.

Energy slumps are also an invitation for you to peek at your overall diet and make sure it's well-rounded and nutrient-packed. Juices and smoothies are your first step toward maximizing your intake of phytonutrients. But a well-rounded diet that incorporates lots of quality foods—greens, veggies, nuts, seeds, whole grains, legumes, healthy fats, and protein—is also an essential way of ensuring your own vitality and strength.

How do I get my partner or kids to try green drinks?

One of the nicest things about smoothies and juices is that the recipes are easy to modify in ways that will be immediately palatable to skeptical newbies, old and young. Start with some super tasty blends, and you'll get them on the leafy green bandwagon, too. For juices, I recommend Sweet Greens (page 138) or Green Me Up (page 130). My Easygoing Green (page 199) and Island Green (page 201) are perfect starter smoothies.

Smoothies and juices can also be treated as go-to indulgences for you and yours. Get your kids into the habit of sipping on fiber-rich, antioxidant-packed smoothies in place of conventional (read: crummy) treats. My Creamsicle smoothie (page 241) has all of

the flavors of the creamy classic frozen dessert, without any of the refined sugars (and it's got a whole lot of vitamin C and healthy fat, to boot). The Mood Lift (page 268) and the Mint Chip Champion (page 229) are perfect alternatives to chocolate milk. If your kids love orange juice, try sneaking in more fruits and veggies by treating them to a diluted Citrus Shine (page 189) or Crimson Dawn (page 155) juice instead.

My kids love the way green smoothies taste, but they just can't get over the green color. What can I do?

Hey, you're not the only one. A lot of grown-ups struggle with the color of green drinks, too. Best solution: use plenty of berries in your smoothies. Not only will they mask the hue, they're also packed with antioxidants. Raw cacao powder will also help. Here's a sneaky trick for kids: pour their smoothie in a colored glass or sippy cup. Poof, no greens here! Another idea is to make it fun. Include your kids in the prep and even let them name the recipes. The "green monster" they participated in creating will probably be more interesting to guzzle than a concoction that's forced upon them.

lip-smackin' recipes

7

JOYFUL
JUICES

THE CLEANSERS

Green is the theme of this whole collection, and these ten juices put it front and center. These are my alkalizing superheroes, the juices you'll want to make again and again to ensure that you're maximizing energy and well-being. Tired? Cranky? Feel a cold coming on? Craving pizza? Allow these green formulas to help you energize and reboot.

mellow green

A perfect juice for when you're craving something green, but not too green. Pears and cucumber are a heavenly duo, and Swiss chard adds some extra alkaline power to the recipe. Keep in mind that Swiss chard leaves can vary dramatically in size; if your leaves are giant (as big as two hands), one single leaf might be enough for the recipe. To vary the flavor, try adding a few sprigs of mint. Voilà!

Makes 2 Servings (16 to 20 Ounces)

2 Bartlett or Bosc pears, cored and seeded

1 cucumber

2 leaves Swiss chard

1   Wash and prep all ingredients.

2   Juice all ingredients.

classic green lemonade

Green lemonade is the Cadillac of juicing recipes. This is my take on the beloved classic. The juice is a little sweet (thanks to the apple) and a little spicy (gracias to the ginger). The natural bitterness of leafy greens is cut by a bright squeeze of lemon. You can use almost any type of leafy green in place of chard or kale. Romaine, baby spinach, collard, bok choy, broccoli—you name it! In fact, I love adding broccoli stems to this recipe. Get creative. This juice is a perfect vehicle for all of your greenest fridge scraps.

Makes 2 Servings (16 to 20 Ounces)

2 stalks celery

1 small cucumber

1 apple, cored and seeded

1-inch piece ginger, peeled

3 leaves Swiss chard or kale

½ lemon, peeled

1   Wash and prep all ingredients.

2   Juice all ingredients.

THE CLEANSERS

soothing green

The name says it all: this is a simple, soothing, and refreshing blend, perfect for showing off the beautiful sweetness
of ripe summer honeydew. Feel free to adjust the mint to
suit your tastes (I like it nice and minty), and to use any
variety of leafy green.

Makes 2 Servings (16 to 20 Ounces)

4 leaves Swiss chard

1 cucumber

3 to 4 tablespoons mint leaves, tightly packed, to taste

3 cups honeydew melon cubes

1   Wash and prep all ingredients.

2   Juice all ingredients.

sweet & sour green

A delicious combination of eye-opening orange and pineapple, mixed with hydrating, alkaline veggies. To make this drink even greener (AKA more powerful), try increasing the spinach or throwing in a fistful of cleansing parsley.

Makes 2 Servings (16 to 20 Ounces)

1 small cucumber

3 stalks celery

1 cup spinach, tightly packed

1 cup pineapple cubes

1 navel orange, peeled

1 Wash and prep all ingredients.

2 Juice all ingredients.

spicy sweetie

This juice recipe is the perfect marriage of zesty and slightly sweet, and it's one of my favorite elixirs. Like most of its fellow green leafy vegetables, arugula is high in vitamin K, which supports bone health. It's also rich in glucosinolates, sulfur-containing compounds that can help release the vegetable's phytochemicals. Arugula is also a lovely addition to green juices because it's got a slightly spicy flavor, especially when it's purchased at the height of freshness. Baby arugula, which is carried in grocery stores year-round, is more mellow.

PRO TIP If this juice isn't quite sweet enough for you, you can try using two pears in place of the tart Granny Smith apples.

Makes 2 Servings (16 to 20 Ounces)

2 cups green cabbage, tightly packed

2 cups arugula, leaves and stems, tightly packed

1 small cucumber

2 large stalks celery

2 Granny Smith apples

1-inch piece ginger, peeled

1　Wash and prep all ingredients.

2　Juice all ingredients.

sweet greens

Fresh watermelon creates an irresistible sweetness that will win over even the stubbornest green juice skeptics. Just keep in mind that juices made with watermelon taste best when the fruit is used in season—underripe, spongy, or dry melons taste a little bitter. You can freeze fresh melon cubes for a few months.

Makes 2 Servings (16 to 20 Ounces)

2½ cups watermelon cubes

2 cups spinach, packed

1 cucumber

¼ lime

1   Wash and prep all ingredients.

2   Juice all ingredients.

THE HEALERS

Plant foods are healing across the board, but the following juices are designed to have a particularly medicinal effect on the body. Whether you're hoping to boost your immunity, soothe your digestion, fight inflammation, or give yourself a dose of protection against chronic disease or hypertension, you're sure to find a suitable elixir here.

root power

This recipe is all about root vegetables: beets, carrots, and daikon radish. Though not a common juice ingredient, daikon is a healthy-spicy addition to any blend. The long, pale white-colored root vegetable is often used in traditional Chinese medicine to help aid digestion and enhance immunity. It's also a mild diuretic, which makes this a handy juice formula when you're feeling a little bloated.

Makes 2 Servings (16 to 20 Ounces)

1 small beet

2 Granny Smith apples, cored and seeded

4 medium carrots

½ small daikon radish (about 5 inches)

1 cucumber

1-inch piece ginger, peeled

1   Wash and prep all ingredients.

2   Juice all ingredients.

immune boost

If your immune system is in SOS mode, then this is the juice for you. Oranges provide loads of vitamin C, which may aid in immune system deficiencies, and carrots have been shown to have a protective effect against multiple cancers (in addition to their famous vision-boosting superpowers!). Turmeric root is a potent anti-inflammatory agent, and if you're starting to get the sniffles, the dash of cayenne will help you sweat them out ASAP. Use one shake if you're sensitive to spice, two to three if you like it red hot.

Makes 2 Servings (16 to 20 Ounces)

4 large carrots
2 navel oranges, peeled
½-inch piece turmeric root
Pinch of cayenne pepper

1   Wash and prep all ingredients.
2   Juice all ingredients.

c bomb

This immunity-boosting beverage is all about vitamin C, which may also help to prevent high blood pressure and high cholesterol. Win-win! I love the purple-haze color that red cabbage lends to this sweet-spicy juice, but green cabbage is a fine replacement if you don't have red on hand.

Makes 2 Servings (16 to 20 Ounces)

1 cucumber
4 stalks celery
2 small apples, cored and seeded
1½ cups red cabbage
1-inch piece of ginger, peeled

1   Wash and prep all ingredients.

2   Juice all ingredients.

ginger aid

This simple and fuss-free blend shows off the signature flavor and healing properties of ginger root. Ginger has long been celebrated for its antinausea properties, so make this your go-to tonic for occasional indigestion. While you sip, you can rest assured that ginger root is also helping to cool inflammation and fight the aging process.

PRO TIP To give this juice even more alkaline power, try throwing in an extra fistful of spinach (or a few leaves of romaine).

Makes 2 Servings (16 to 20 Ounces)

1½ cups spinach
1 large cucumber-
2 stalks celery
1 large pear, cored and seeded
1-inch piece ginger, peeled

1   Wash and prep all ingredients.
2   Juice all ingredients.

crimson dawn

Good morning, gorgeous! It's time to strut your stuff. This juice is a perfect wakeup call. I love the combination of zippy citrus and grounding root vegetables. You'll also get a hit of red bell pepper, which is an incredible source of vitamin C. Forget those cold-fighting powders and lozenges, and try a sip of this immune-boosting elixir instead. Now go kick some butt!

Makes 2 Servings (16 to 20 Ounces)

4 medium carrots

1 medium beet

1 large navel orange, peeled

1 red bell pepper, stem and seeds removed

2 stalks celery

¾–1 inch piece ginger, peeled

1   Wash and prep all ingredients.

2   Juice all ingredients.

THE HEALERS

tummy tamer

Fennel has long been known as a balm for all sorts of digestive woes, from indigestion and heartburn to bloating and irregularity. It's thought to stimulate bile secretion, which can help keep digestion running smoothly and allow you to assimilate your food efficiently.

In this refreshing and mildly sweet juice, fennel meets ginger—another belly-soothing superstar—and hydrating cucumber. The combination of ingredients can help to keep nausea and bloating at bay. This is a perfect elixir to sip before or after a heavy meal.

Makes 2 Servings (16 to 20 Ounces)

½ small head fennel (about ½ cup)
1 large or 2 small cucumbers
2 stalks celery
⅛ cup mint, leaves and stems, tightly packed
2 apples
1-inch piece ginger, peeled

1   Wash and prep all ingredients.
2   Juice all ingredients.

the sicilian

This vegetable-packed elixir first appeared in *Crazy Sexy Kitchen*, and it won us over with its spicy and satisfying taste. It's hearty and savory, just the recipe you'll want when your tummy's rumbling. The celery in this juice provides phthalide, a phytochemical that can help to relax the smooth muscles of the arteries and lower blood pressure. The garlic provides not only a zesty taste, but also plenty of immunity-boosting antibacterial properties. As the Italians would say, "Bevi!"

PRO TIP Be sure to remove all seeds from the jalapeño pepper before running it through your juicer. Most of the zing is housed in the seeds, and they can overpower your juice if they happen to slip in!

Makes 2 Servings (16 to 20 Ounces)

6 medium carrots

3 large tomatoes

2 red bell peppers

2 cloves garlic

4 stalks celery

1 cup watercress

1 cup loosely packed spinach

1 red jalapeño, seeded (optional)

1   Wash and prep all ingredients.

2   Juice all ingredients.

THE BOOSTERS

These juices are on the sweeter side, which means that they're perfect for a healthy energy boost. Struggling with the 3 P.M. lull? Hoping to make a fruity and refreshing summer drink for a get-together with friends? Allow these juices to lift your spirits. The boosters are also a great option for those of us who are a little skittish about the taste of greens.

If you love these energizing recipes, but you're being mindful of the sweetness in your juices, simply follow my tips on page 53 for reducing the sugar content of juices or smoothies.

orange uplift

This sunny, sweet, refreshing juice is a wonderful morning wake-up call. There's no actual orange in here, but cantaloupe and carrots help to create a vibrant color. Cantaloupe is a superstar source of vitamins A and C, both of which help to keep your skin and eyes healthy and your immune system strong. Cantaloupe is also rich in potassium, which aids in hydration and helps to keep your blood pressure steady.

PRO TIP To make this mixture slightly less sweet, try substituting one cucumber for the carrots.

Makes 2 Servings (16 to 20 Ounces)

2 cups cantaloupe cubes

2 medium carrots

4 stalks celery

½ head romaine lettuce (about 8 to 10 leaves)

1   Wash and prep all ingredients.

2   Juice all ingredients.

blueberry lemon-aid

Conventional lemonade recipes are packed with added sugars (and the bottled ones have some not-so-savory additives and preservatives, too). This mixture evokes the beloved taste of freshly made lemonade, but it's infused with body-boosting ingredients. The cucumbers create a hydrating base for the juice, while apples provide a lovely sweetness that's not too sugary. The fresh blueberries add age-defying antioxidants and help give the drink a gorgeous purple color.

PRO TIP This is another great recipe to keep handy for summer entertaining, or to offer kids as a more nutritious spin on a favorite childhood classic!

Makes 2 Servings (16 to 20 Ounces)

2 small cucumbers

1 cup blueberries

2 Granny Smith apples

¼ lemon, peeled

3 tablespoons mint leaves, tightly packed

1   Wash and prep all ingredients.

2   Juice all ingredients.

pretty in pink

This electric pink juice is a beet lover's dream! The combination of pineapple and Granny Smith apple is as delightfully tart as it is sweet. Plus, ginger adds a little heat to the mixture. To lessen the sweetness of the juice, try substituting a cucumber for the apple and adding a handful of mild greens, like spinach or romaine.

Makes 2 Servings (16 to 20 Ounces)

2 cups pineapple, cubed
1 Granny Smith apple, cored and seeded
1 medium beet
1-inch piece ginger, peeled

1   Wash and prep all ingredients.
2   Juice all ingredients.

herbal elixer

This cheery drink is an ode to summer's most beloved
ingredients, from cucumber to pineapple to fresh basil.
I recommend making it seasonally, when your herbs and
fruits are at the peak of freshness. Basil contains tons of
flavonoids that can help to protect your skin against aging
and UV damage.

Makes 2 Servings (16 to 20 Ounces)

1 large cucumber

2½ cups pineapple cubes

¼ cup basil, leaves and stems, tightly packed

¼ cup cilantro or parsley, leaves and stems, tightly packed

⅛ cup mint leaves, tightly packed

4 stalks kale

1   Wash and prep all ingredients.

2   Juice all ingredients.

blushing beauty

Peaches and yum! This juice is both herbal and fruity, a light and unusual combination. You'll be delighted at the taste (and dusty rose color) that strawberries and peaches lend to the elixir. You can also feel good about the fact that this juice is like a liquid prescription for beautiful skin! It's incredibly high in vitamin C, which helps us to form collagen (an important structural component of strong skin) and fight off free radicals. Peaches are also high in beta-carotene, which is associated with cell repair.

PRO TIP You can substitute other summer berries, like blackberries or raspberries, for the strawberries in this recipe.

Makes 2 Servings (16 to 20 Ounces)

1 large cucumber

2 large peaches, pitted

3 cups strawberries

2 tablespoons basil leaves, tightly packed

1   Wash and prep all ingredients.

2   Juice all ingredients.

feelin' hot, hot, hot

Spice up your juice routine with this unusual blend of mellow honeydew and spicy jalapeño. I love to drink this one as a cocktail on hot summer nights; the cilantro is a wonderfully refreshing addition. As always, adjust the jalapeño to suit your taste (and tolerance for heat!).

PRO TIP If you don't have ripe honeydew on hand, try watermelon instead.

Makes 2 Servings (16 to 20 Ounces)

1½ cups honeydew melon cubes

2 leaves kale

¼ cup cilantro, leaves and stems, tightly packed

1 large cucumber

1 to 2 jalapeño peppers, seeds removed

1 Wash and prep all ingredients.

2 Juice all ingredients.

pucker up

This sassy breakfast blend is a fire hose of sunshine — and it's anti-inflammatory, antibacterial, and immune boosting to boot! Citrus and ginger are a delightful combination, and I love the balance of tart grapefruit and sweet oranges. Lemon gives the juice an extra dose of pucker (and an alkaline boost, too).

Makes 2 Servings (16 to 20 Ounces)

1 pink grapefruit, peeled

3 navel oranges, peeled

½-inch piece turmeric root

1-inch piece ginger, peeled

¼ lemon, peeled

1   Wash and prep all ingredients.

2   Juice all ingredients.

bloat buster

Belly bloat got you down? Then it's time for a sip of this refreshing, clean juice. It's a honeydew lover's delight, featuring a mixture of fresh melon and a gaggle of greens. The parsley and dandelion greens act as a gentle and natural diuretic, helping you to shed water weight and feel less puffy. Make this your cocktail of choice when PMS calls, when you've been too busy to hydrate properly, or when you simply need to feel refreshed.

Makes 2 Servings (16 to 20 Ounces)

6 leaves dandelion greens

1 large cucumber

2 large leaves Swiss chard

⅛ cup parsley, leaves and stems, tightly packed

2 cups honeydew melon cubes

1   Wash and prep all ingredients.

2   Juice all ingredients.

citrus shine

Pucker, power, pow! This delightful formula will help kick-start your day with a medley of sweet and sour flavors. Tart apple, orange, and lemon are mellowed out by sweet kiwi and the hydrating cucumber.

Makes 2 Servings (16 to 20 Ounces)

1 kiwi

1 medium apple, cored and seeded

1 navel orange, peeled

2 cucumbers

½ lemon

1   Wash and prep all ingredients.

2   Juice all ingredients.

hello hydration

I absolutely adore this combination of three simple ingredients—it's like a summery Italian salad in a glass! Watermelon lends irresistible sweetness to the mixture, while the cucumber and the savory addition of basil mellow it out. You'll want to make this juice when watermelon is ripe—so it's worth waiting until summer. Serve it to friends at cookouts, garden parties, or brunches, and be prepared to smile at their ooh's and ah's.

Makes 2 Servings (16 to 20 Ounces)

1 large cucumber

3 cups watermelon

¼ cup basil, leaves and stems, tightly packed

1 Wash and prep all ingredients.

2 Juice all ingredients.

fatigue fighter

This vivacious juice will pick you up and get you going with a touch of sweetness from pears and grapes and hints of tartness from the lime. Pears are rich in vitamin B2, which plays a crucial role in energy production and helps us metabolize iron—an important nutrient in maintaining energy levels. Some studies suggest that grapes may help to boost cognitive function (always useful!). Make this your go-to juice cocktail for those mornings when you need a little extra brain and body power.

Makes 2 Servings (16 to 20 Ounces)

8 leaves romaine
1 cup spinach, tightly packed
2 stalks celery
1 pear
1½ cups grapes, green or red
¼ lime, peeled

1 Wash and prep all ingredients.
2 Juice all ingredients.

THE BEAUTIFIERS

SCRUMPTIOUS
SMOOTHIES

easygoing green

The name says it all. This green smoothie is easy to love.
It's also super hydrating, thanks to the addition of coconut
water, and chock-full of healthy fats from the avocado.
The more avocado you add, the thicker the texture will be,
so feel free to add up to half a Hass avocado if you'd like
something a little thicker (see my tips for storing leftover
avocado halves on page 74).

Makes 2 Servings (16 to 20 Ounces)

1 large banana, frozen

1 cup mango cubes, frozen

2 cups coconut water (see page 131 for my favorite brands)

¼ Hass avocado

¼ cup curly parsley, stems and leaves, tightly packed

1 cup kale, leaves only, tightly packed

1   Wash and prep all ingredients.

2   Blend and serve.

calming greens

This smoothie is a go-to in our home. I love the refreshing addition of cilantro and mint, and avocado creates a luscious texture. If you don't happen to have grapes handy, try kiwi or honeydew melon in their place. If you do have grapes, oh boy, you're gonna be happy.

Makes 2 Servings (16 to 20 Ounces)

1 banana, frozen

1 cup green grapes

¼ Hass avocado

⅓ cup cilantro, leaves and stems, tightly packed

¼ cup fresh mint leaves, tightly packed

1 cup spinach, tightly packed

1¼ cups water

1   Wash and prep all ingredients.

2   In a high-speed blender, blend all ingredients. Serve.

peachy green

This recipe was inspired by my favorite summer fruit stand—the peaches are out-of-control delicious and juicy. I buy one for my bike ride home and the rest for smoothies! In this blend, peaches and banana meet heart-healthy flax seeds and a creamy base of cashew hemp milk.

Makes 2 Servings (16 to 20 Ounces)

1 large banana, frozen

1 cup peaches, peeled, pitted, and cut into chunks or slices (fresh or frozen)

1 tablespoon flax seeds, ground

1½ cups cashew hemp milk (page 276) or nondairy milk of choice

1 cup Swiss chard, washed, stems removed, and torn into pieces (about 2 large leaves), tightly packed

1   Wash and prep all ingredients.

2   Blend and serve.

THE pH WARRIORS

detox darling

If detoxing could taste this good all the time, we'd all be fit as fiddles! The sprouts give this blend an earthy, nutty flavor, which is balanced perfectly by sweet pear and banana. Sunflower sprouts are one of the most nutritious sprouts around, featuring plenty of protein, B vitamins, and zinc, the latter of which is essential for immune function, while the leafy greens support your body's natural detoxification processes.

Makes 2 Servings (16 to 20 Ounces)

½ cup dandelion greens, tightly packed
1 cup baby spinach, tightly packed
⅓ cup sunflower sprouts, tightly packed
½ large or 1 small pear, cored and seeded
1 banana, frozen
1½ cups almond milk (page 274) or nondairy milk of choice

1   Wash and prep all ingredients.
2   Blend till smooth and serve.

THE pH WARRIORS

granny smith apple pie

Who doesn't love a good ole slice of apple pie? Well, this smoothie is the next best thing. It's sweet, a little tart, and the cinnamon evokes Grandma's favorite dessert perfectly.

APPLES AND PEARS IN SMOOTHIES

Apples and pears make wonderful additions to smoothies, adding a thick, almost "fluffy" texture to the mix, along with sweetness. If you'd like to add extra fiber to your smoothie, then leave the skin on the fruit. If you'd like your blend to have a smoother texture, then you'll want to peel your apples or pears after you core and seed them.

Makes 2 Servings (20 to 24 Ounces)

1 banana, frozen

1 Granny Smith apple, cored, peeled, and seeded

1½ cups kale, leaves only, tightly packed

1½ cups pumpkin seed milk (page 288) or nondairy milk of choice

¼ teaspoon cinnamon

1 pitted Medjool date (optional)

1 Wash and prep all ingredients.

2 Blend and serve.

THE BODY BOOSTERS

Smoothies are incredibly powerful vehicles for optimum nutrition. The following blends have been designed to help you boost your daily intake of some of the nutrients our bodies' need most dearly: iron, calcium, fatty acids, and protein. If you're being nagged with the "where do you get your protein" question, friends, you can rest assured that these particular recipes are designed to give you a meal-worthy protein boost.

popeye

Be strong to the finish with this vibrantly colored, delicious green blend. Spinach wins special favor in the vegetable kingdom for its incredible store of anti-inflammatory and cancer-fighting flavonoids, and it's an excellent source of iron. Meanwhile, the mango in this recipe provides 100 percent of your recommended daily dose of superstar antioxidant vitamin C. This smoothie tastes mildly tropical, and it's one of my go-to green blends.

Makes 2 Servings (20 to 24 Ounces)

1 banana, frozen

¾ cup mango cubes, frozen

2 cups spinach, tightly packed

1 teaspoon chia seeds

1⅔ cups pumpkin seed milk (page 288) or nondairy milk of choice

1   Wash and prep all ingredients.

2   Blend and serve.

THE BODY BOOSTERS

sesame superhero

You'll be fighting off foes with this powerful potion. It showcases all of the nutritional superpowers of the humble sesame seed: iron, protein, and calcium. It also contains tons of potassium and vitamins K, A, and C, thanks to banana and a heaping cup of collard greens. Raisins, which are used to sweeten this smoothie in place of the usual Medjool dates, are a great and often overlooked source of iron—plus, they're packed with belly-friendly fiber, too.

Makes 2 Servings (16 to 20 Ounces)

1 cup collard greens, cut into ribbons, tightly packed

1 large banana, frozen

1 tablespoon tahini

1½ cups sesame seed milk (page 289) or nondairy milk of choice

⅛ cup raisins, packed

½ teaspoon vanilla extract or powder

1   Wash and prep all ingredients.

2   Blend till smooth and serve.

body builder

This protein-packed smoothie is my go-to meal before or after a workout. Peanut butter and hemp seeds help to build and repair muscle, while the kale keeps things mean, green, and loaded with minerals like calcium and iron. Substitute any of your favorite nut milks for the almond milk in this recipe; cashew hemp milk (page 276) will give you an added dose of protein, too.

Makes 2 Servings (20 to 24 Ounces)

2 small bananas, frozen

2 cups almond milk (page 274) or nondairy milk of choice

2 tablespoons hemp seeds

2 tablespoons all-natural peanut butter

2 cups kale, leaves only, tightly packed

1 pitted Medjool date

1 Wash and prep all ingredients.

2 Blend and serve.

sweet sustenance

If you like oatmeal cookies as much as I do, you'll love this recipe. Rolled oats add a thick creamy texture and are also rich in soluble fiber, which can help you feel full for a super long time. The recipe gets a flavor boost from ground cinnamon and a touch of sweetness from lucuma powder.

PRO TIP Lucuma is a fruit native to Peru, and powder derived from the fruit has a mildly sweet flavor that hovers somewhere between butterscotch and vanilla. As an added bonus, it can be used as a low-glycemic sweetener. You can find the powder at health-food stores and online; I like Navitas Naturals and Sunfoods brands.

Makes 2 Servings (20 to 24 Ounces)

1 banana, frozen

⅓ cup rolled oats

2 tablespoons almond butter

¼ teaspoon cinnamon

1 tablespoon lucuma powder

1½ cups cashew hemp milk (page 276) or nondairy milk of choice

1 Wash and prep all ingredients.

2 Blend and serve.

berry protein power

Berries and chocolate are like Fred and Ginger—a beloved pair. Hemp seeds and kale make this smoothie especially nutrient dense, plus the combination of banana and almond milk make it oh-so-creamy.

Makes 2 Servings (20 to 24 Ounces)

1 large banana, frozen

1 cup blueberries, frozen

1½ cups almond milk (page 274) or nondairy milk of choice

2 tablespoons hemp seeds

2 tablespoons cacao nibs

1 cup kale, leaves only, tightly packed

1   Wash and prep all ingredients.

2   Blend and serve.

mint chip champion

If you like classic Girl Scout cookies, you'll love this smoothie. It's a minty, chocolatey bonanza! It's also packed with anti-inflammatory spinach, antioxidant rich cacao nibs, and my creamy, protein-packed cashew hemp milk. It even has a spunky, mint green color and loads of leafy green goodness.

PRO TIP If you don't have cacao nibs at home, don't sweat it. They add some delightful texture to the smoothie, but one tablespoon of regular ole cocoa powder (or raw cacao powder, if that's what you've got) is a fine substitute.

Makes 2 Servings (20 to 24 Ounces)

1½ cups spinach, tightly packed

2 bananas, frozen

1 to 2 pitted Medjool dates

2 tablespoons mint leaves

1½ tablespoons cacao nibs

2 cups cashew hemp milk (page 276), or nondairy milk of choice

1   Wash and prep all ingredients.

2   Blend till smooth and serve.

watermelon quencher

Don't let the simplicity of this blend fool you. The combination of mint, watermelon, and banana is divine, and the drink is a powerful boost for your skin and energy. Watermelon is about 92 percent water, which—combined with the electrolytes from coconut water in this recipe—will help to keep you hydrated no matter how hot the day. As a beautifying added bonus, watermelon is also a great source of lycopene, which helps to protect against free radical damage and aging.

Makes 2 Servings (20 to 24 Ounces)

1 banana, frozen

½ cucumber

1 cup watermelon cubes

1¼ cups coconut water

1 tablespoon mint leaves

1 Wash and prep all ingredients.

2 Blend and serve.

strawberry fields

This refreshing blend is one of my favorites from *Crazy Sexy Kitchen*. I love the way that lemon zest and orange brighten the smoothie (and infuse it with immunity boosting vitamin C). Strawberries also contribute vitamin C (a whopping 150 percent of your recommended daily allowance per serving) along with folic acid, which can help to regulate blood pressure and prevent anemia. Finally, these gorgeous berries provide the phytonutrient ellagic acid, which is thought to help keep the collagen in your skin healthy. Cheers!

Makes 2 Servings (24 to 30 Ounces)

3 cups cashew hemp milk (page 276) or nondairy milk of choice

2 cups fresh strawberries

1 tablespoon lemon zest

1 small orange, peeled

1 small banana

1½ cups loosely packed spinach

1 Wash and prep all ingredients.

2 Blend till smooth and serve.

chocolate avocado

One of my favorite raw food desserts is chocolate avocado pudding (don't be grossed out; it's actually a surprisingly delicious treat). I like to think of this smoothie as the sip-worthy version of that fabulous recipe. This is a perfect goodie when chocolate cravings pay a visit!

Makes 2 Servings (20 to 24 Ounces)

2 small bananas, frozen

1 to 2 pitted Medjool dates

1½ tablespoons cacao powder

¼ Hass avocado

1¾ cup almond milk (page 274) or nondairy milk of choice

½ teaspoon vanilla extract

1 cup baby spinach, tightly packed

1   Wash and prep all ingredients.

2   Blend till smooth and serve.

creamsicle

This smoothie pays homage to my favorite Popsicle—
without the corn syrup and artificial flavors. You'll be
amazed at how well it captures the sweet, refreshing taste
we all remember, and unlike the original childhood treat,
it's brimming with vitamin C, potassium, and healthy fats.
What's not to love?

1 orange, peeled, pith removed, and cut into quarters

1 banana, frozen

½ teaspoon vanilla extract or powder

⅛ cup raw cashews

1½ cups cashew hemp milk (page 276) or nondairy milk of choice

1   Wash and prep all ingredients.

2   Blend till smooth and serve.

deep blue beauty

Hey, gorgeous, I bet I'm not the first person to tell you about acai, a super berry that hails from South and Central America. Acai is full of powerful antioxidants, as well as complete proteins. Unfortunately, a lot of the commercial juices and bottled beverages that feature acai are packed with artificial ingredients or sweeteners.

PRO TIP You can purchase unsweetened acai smoothie packs from the Sambazon brand (just check labels for the unsweetened flavor). Acai has a rich, unusual, and only mildly sweet flavor, so it's helpful to whirl it up with sweet bananas and berries. I like to use my creamy Brazil nut milk (page 287) in this smoothie, but commercial nondairy milk is a fine substitute if you don't have any on hand.

Makes 2 Servings (16 to 20 Ounces)

1 banana, frozen

½ pack (50 grams, or 1¼ ounces) unsweetened frozen acai pulp

½ cup blueberries, frozen

1½ cups spinach, packed

1 tablespoon coconut oil or coconut butter

2 teaspoons raw cacao powder

1 pitted Medjool date

1½ cups Brazil nut milk (page 287)

1 teaspoon spirulina or blue-green algae

1 Wash and prep all ingredients.

2 Blend and serve.

raspberry revitalizer

This delicious smoothie will make you feel as though you're drinking dessert through a straw—but it'll also help to boost your vitality with healthful fatty acids and greens.

PRO TIP Coconut butter adds a wonderful creaminess and subtly decadent flavor to smoothies—a nice departure from almond or peanut butter, if those are your go-to's. It can be a little tricky to find, but you should be able to get your hands on some at most health-food stores or online.

Makes 2 Servings (20 to 24 Ounces)

1 cup kale, tightly packed

1 cup raspberries, frozen

1 banana, frozen

1 tablespoon coconut butter or coconut oil

½ teaspoon vanilla extract

1¾ cups Brazil nut milk (page 287) or nondairy milk of choice

1   Wash and prep all ingredients.

2   Blend till smooth and serve.

hangover helper

Did ya party a little too hardy? Kiss that headache good-bye with this little helper. This delicious blend features tons of hydrating foods to help get you back on your feet—including potassium-rich banana, cucumber, and coconut water. It also features some healthy fats in the form of creamy avocado to lift your energy levels, and plenty of leafy greens and lemons to help your body cleanse and detox.

Makes 2 Servings (16 to 20 Ounces)

½ banana, frozen

1 cup honeydew melon, cubed

½ cucumber, peeled

½ cup watercress, leaves and top parts of stems, tightly packed

1 cup spinach, tightly packed

2 tablespoons parsley, tightly packed

½-inch piece ginger, peeled

2 teaspoons lemon juice

¼ Hass avocado

1½ cups coconut water

1   Wash and prep all ingredients.

2   Blend till smooth and serve.

cherry chocolate bliss

Love chocolate-covered cherries? Then this smoothie is for you. I'm cuckoo for the combination of raw cacao, creamy avocado, almond milk, and sweet cherries—it's like dessert in a glass, in the best of ways. I also love that the smoothie is bursting with anthocyanins, plant pigments that give cherries their beautiful color and help keep our skin strong (while also warding off inflammation).

And because the best desserts are as healthy as they are delicious, I've thrown in some nutrient-rich leafy greens in the form of spinach (though you're welcome to use your favorite green here instead!).

Makes 2 Servings (16 to 20 Ounces)

1½ cups spinach, tightly packed

1 cup cherries, frozen

1 banana, frozen

¼ Hass avocado

1 tablespoon raw cacao powder

1½ cups almond milk (page 274) or nondairy milk of choice

1 Wash and prep all ingredients.

2 Blend and serve.

THE SUPERHEROES

The following blends are unexpected and invigorating. They're also functional. Many of them are infused with superfoods, like maca, cacao, or matcha powder. These unique ingredients can help our bodies with repair, energy production, healing, hormone balance, and a host of other vital functions (for more on superfoods, see page 85).

These blends cover a vast array of texture, taste, and use: some, like my "Quick Recovery" smoothie, are light and fruity, while others, like my "All Day Energy" shake, are creamy and rich. My hope is that they'll inspire you to think outside the smoothie box!

hot flash healer

Lady, no need to open a window in the dead of winter—maca to the rescue! In this smoothie, hormone-balancing maca tangos with the natural phytoestrogens in flax seed, which are thought to help relieve menopause symptoms.

Makes 2 Servings (16 to 20 Ounces)

1½ cups strawberries, frozen

1 apple, cored and seeded

1 tablespoon flax seeds, ground

1 teaspoon maca powder

1½ cups macadamia maple milk (page 277) or nondairy milk of choice

1   Wash and prep all ingredients.

2   Blend and serve.

I don't know abo

'70s. Back in my gro
ing bras for their n
thirteen or fourtee
"period party" cele
nese restaurant (
kids as young as
son–stacked rug
it's dangerous.

Steroids an
beef, pork, an
make the an
hormones?
year round.
mones so s
lactating—
such an u

She's
growth
duction
hormo
3, is li
tory,
inter

hormone helper

Our Crazy Sexy hormones are in flux all throughout our lifecycles: for ladies, this includes puberty, childbirth, and menopause. While hormonal changes can often create bodily ouchies, nature graciously provides certain nutrients that can help to lessen the dreaded aches, pains, and hot flashes.

PRO TIP Phytoestrogens, a class of phytonutrients found in soy, flax, and sesame seeds, can gently mimic the effects of estrogen in the body, helping to lessen the symptoms of PMS and menopause. You'll find plenty of them, along with libido-enhancing maca, in this creamy smoothie. On page 77, you'll find instructions for how to open a young Thai coconut. You can also use a frozen brand, like Exotic Superfoods. If you don't have a source for young Thai coconut, try using ¼ avocado in this recipe instead.

Makes 2 Servings (20 to 24 Ounces)

1 banana, frozen

½ cup blueberries, frozen

½ cup young Thai coconut meat

1¾ cups Brazil nut milk (page 287) or nondairy milk of choice

1 teaspoon flax seeds, ground

1 teaspoon maca

1 cup spinach, tightly packed

1   Wash and prep all ingredients.

2   Blend and serve.

digestive fire

All these ingredients add up to awesome. In the Ayurvedic tradition, the body's digestive power is imagined as fire, or Agni. Stoke your digestive furnace with this smoothie, which features belly-soothing mint, inflammation-taming ginger, electrolyte-balancing banana, and the natural digestive, pineapple. Pineapple is an excellent source of the enzyme bromelain, which digests protein. It may give your digestive system a powerful boost. Some studies have suggested that bromelain may help to ease symptoms of osteoarthritis as well.

Makes 2 Servings (16 to 20 Ounces)

1 banana, frozen

1 cup pineapple chunks, frozen

1½ cups coconut water

1 cup kale, tightly packed

2 tablespoons fresh mint, chopped

¾-inch piece of ginger, peeled

1   Wash and prep all ingredients.

2   Blend and serve.

morning jolt

Okay, so this smoothie can be a wee bit more demand-
ing, because it involves making fresh carrot juice and
then blending it into a (blissful) smoothie. If the idea of
using two appliances sends you running, then just keep
this smoothie on the back burner for a leisurely weekend
morning. Once you try it, I promise you won't mind the
extra elbow grease; the combination of carrot, banana, and
ginger is ah-mazing. Plus, a boost of maca and cashews
means that this smoothie can sustain your energy all the
way to lunchtime.

Makes 2 Servings (16 to 20 Ounces)

1 cup carrot juice

½ cup coconut water

1 large banana, frozen

½-inch piece of ginger, peeled

¼ cup cashews

1 teaspoon maca powder

1 Wash and prep all ingredients.

2 Blend and serve.

all day energy

This smoothie is creamy, filling, and designed to help keep your energy levels stable and strong throughout the day. Matcha is a form of stone-ground green tea leaves. It's thought to have all of the antioxidant benefits of green tea, but in a more concentrated form. In addition to its energy enhancing qualities, matcha is associated with mood regulation, increased metabolism, and antioxidant power. It makes a wonderful addition to smoothies (especially if you're trying to kick the coffee habit).

PRO TIP In this blend, matcha plays deliciously well with avocado, banana, and vanilla. I recommend using homemade almond milk or cashew hemp milk in this smoothie if you can; they really enhance the taste!

Makes 2 Servings (16 to 20 Ounces)

1 teaspoon matcha green tea powder

¼ ripe avocado

1 banana, frozen

1½ cups almond milk (page 274) or cashew hemp milk (page 276)

2 teaspoons maple syrup or 1 pitted Medjool date

½ teaspoon vanilla extract

1 Wash and prep all ingredients.

2 Blend till smooth and serve.

THE SUPERHEROES

antioxidant boost

This smoothie is an antioxidant, free-radical busting, inflammation-fighting superhero! You could literally serve it in a cape and tights. Goji berries, which have been used for years in Traditional Chinese Medicine, are a complete source of protein and provide iron, zinc, and vitamin C along with their incredible phytonutrient stores. The catechin EGCG, which is abundant in matcha powder, is associated with a reduced risk of cancer (and the little boost of caffeine will perk you up, too). See, I told ya it was a superhero in disguise. To your health!

Makes 2 Servings (16 to 20 Ounces)

1 cup mixed berries, frozen
½ cup blueberries, frozen
¼ cup goji berries
1½ cups cashew hemp milk (page 276) or nondairy milk of choice
½ teaspoon matcha green tea powder
1 cup spinach, tightly packed

1   Wash and prep all ingredients.

2   Blend and serve.

brain booster

Blueberries aren't just a delicious way to sweeten your smoothies (and give them a gorgeous, deep blue hue). They're also powerful brain boosters. In clinical studies, blueberries have been associated with increased cognitive function, including memory improvement, and they may also help to protect your brain from oxidative stress, lessening the risk of Alzheimer's disease and dementia. The omega-3 fatty acids in walnuts are also associated with cognitive protection, and a possible mood lift: omega-3's are thought to help fight depression. Who knew there could be so much power in your glass? (You did!).

Makes 2 Servings (16 to 20 Ounces)

½ banana, frozen

1½ cups blueberries, frozen

1½ cups almond milk (page 274) or nondairy milk of choice

2 tablespoons walnuts, chopped

1 cup kale, leaves only, tightly packed

½ teaspoon cinnamon, ground

1   Wash and prep all ingredients.

2   Blend and serve.

THE SUPERHEROES

ginger chia supercharger

Supercharger is right. This smoothie packs in protein from chia seeds, almond milk, almond butter, and kale, which makes it a perfect go-to before or after a workout. I love the combination of ginger, mango, and almond—it tastes decadent but fruity and uplifting at the same time.

PRO TIP If you don't have mango, substitute pineapple or extra banana instead. Or, for a very different—but also very delicious—blend, try swapping blueberries for mango.

Makes 2 Servings (20 to 24 Ounces)

1 cup kale, leaves only, tightly packed

1 banana, frozen

1 cup mango, frozen and cubed

½-inch piece ginger, peeled

1 teaspoon chia seeds

1 tablespoon almond butter

1¾ cups almond milk (page 274) or nondairy milk of choice

1   Wash and prep all ingredients.

2   Blend till smooth and serve.

THE SUPERHEROES

9

RADIANT NUT AND SEED MILKS

basic nut milk formula

I've listed quite a few nut milk recipes in this chapter, but I also wanted to give you a basic recipe that will work with many different nuts. Here's a basic formula to get you started.

PRO TIP I like to use Medjool dates, which contain minerals and antioxidants along with natural sugar, but maple syrup, coconut syrup, and yacon syrup also work well as sweeteners.

Yields 4 Cups

1 cup nuts, soaked overnight and rinsed

3 to 4 cups filtered water (depending on how creamy a blend you'd like)

A pinch of salt

Sweetener to taste

1   Blend the mixture thoroughly, until it looks totally uniform and frothy (a few minutes). To strain, you can use a double layer of cheesecloth or a nut milk bag. Nut milk bags are a great and inexpensive investment (they retail for about $8 to $10 on Amazon, at Bed Bath & Beyond, or at your local health food store), and they make it even easier to create perfectly smooth nut milks at home. Hold your nut milk bag or your cheesecloth over a large bowl, and pour the unstrained nut milk through. Use the bag or cloth to squeeze the contents thoroughly, making sure to extract every drop! Store your nut milk in an airtight container in the fridge for up to 3 or 4 days.

chocolate almond milk

Your inner kiddo will go nuts for this milk. Grab some graham crackers and cuddle up with your books as you sip on this wonderful, dairy-free treat.

PRO TIP You don't have to use cacao powder in this recipe—cocoa powder will work, too—but cacao powder tends to be more potent than cocoa powder, and I love the way its bold flavor comes to life in this recipe. I also like to add a little bit of cinnamon, but feel free to leave it out if you prefer your almond milk on the super traditional side.

Yields 3½ to 4 Cups

1 cup almonds, soaked for 8 hours

2 to 3 pitted Medjool dates

¼ teaspoon salt

4 cups water

2 tablespoons cacao powder

¼ teaspoon cinnamon (optional)

1 In a high-speed blender, blend the almonds, dates, salt, and water till totally smooth.

2 Create a large, double layer of cheesecloth and hold it over a large mixing bowl, or hold a nut milk bag over a large mixing bowl. Pour the almond milk through the cheesecloth or bag and squeeze thoroughly. You can compost or discard the nut pulp.

3 Transfer strained almond milk back to your blender. Add the cacao and cinnamon, if using. Blend till smooth.

4 Transfer the nut milk to an airtight container. It will keep in the fridge for about 3 days.

cashew chai milk

"Get your chai on!" as Oprah would say. This recipe is sweet, spicy, and all-around divine. It's wonderful blended up with fresh banana and greens, and it also pairs well with tropical fruits. For a creamy evening treat, warm a cup over the stovetop, sprinkle with cinnamon, and sip to your heart's content.

Yields 3¾ Cups

1 cup raw cashews, soaked for 2 hours, rinsed, and drained

½-inch piece ginger, peeled

1 teaspoon cinnamon

¼ teaspoon cardamom

¼ teaspoon salt

2 to 3 tablespoons maple syrup

3¼ cups water

1   In a high-speed blender, blend all ingredients till creamy and smooth. Store in an airtight container for up to three days in the fridge.

turmeric milk

Turmeric in your milk? Are you cray cray? Yes! Don't tell the other nut milks, but this recipe is my favorite. Once upon a time, the only thing I knew about turmeric was that it had a brilliant yellow-orange color, which makes it a perfect addition to tofu scrambles. But with the right combination of supporting spices and sweetness, this turmeric twist is out of sight. Plus, it contains incredible anti-inflammatory properties. Turmeric milk can be served cold or warmed on the stovetop for an after-dinner treat.

Yields 3½ Cups

3 cups almond milk (page 274)

4 ounces canned coconut milk (full or reduced fat)

1½ teaspoons turmeric powder or 1-inch fresh turmeric root, peeled

½-inch piece ginger, peeled

½ teaspoon cinnamon

¼ teaspoon cardamom

2 tablespoons maple syrup

1   Blend all ingredients together in a blender till smooth. Store in an airtight container in the fridge for up to 4 days.

green milk

I know what you're thinking: green milk?! It may seem like a nutty idea, but why not infuse your go-to almond milk with a little green goodness? This milk is perfect for sipping, and if you use it in green smoothies, you'll be doubling up on plant power.

PRO TIP To make the milk, follow my basic almond milk formula, adding kale and spinach in the blending step. Then you strain and serve as you normally would. The resulting mixture is sweet and creamy, and even though you'll barely taste the veggies, your body will thank you for them!

Yields 4 Cups

2 leaves kale, stems removed

2 cups baby spinach, packed

1 cup almonds, soaked for 8 hours

2 to 3 pitted Medjool dates

¼ teaspoon salt

1 teaspoon vanilla extract

4 cups water

1 In a high-speed blender, blend all ingredients till totally smooth.

2 Create a large, double layer of cheesecloth and hold it over a large mixing bowl, or hold a nut milk bag over a large mixing bowl. Pour the green milk through the cheesecloth or bag and squeeze thoroughly. You can compost or discard the nut pulp. Transfer the nut milk to an airtight container. It will keep in the fridge for about 3 days.

brazil nut milk

Talk about luxurious. If you could drink cashmere, this is how it would taste. Brazil nuts are an excellent source of selenium, a mineral with strong antioxidant properties. Groovy, no? More important, they make a super creamy and delicious nut milk. I use this one whenever I want a particularly rich flavor and texture.

Yields 3½ to 4 Cups

1 cup Brazil nuts, soaked for 4 hours

2 to 3 pitted Medjool dates

¼ teaspoon salt

1½ teaspoon vanilla extract or the seeds of 1 vanilla bean, scraped

4 cups water

1   In a high-speed blender, blend all ingredients till totally smooth.

2   Create a large, double layer of cheesecloth and hold it over a large mixing bowl, or hold a nut milk bag over a large mixing bowl. Pour the Brazil nut milk through the cheesecloth or bag and squeeze thoroughly. You can compost or discard the nut pulp. Transfer the nut milk to an airtight container. It will keep in the fridge for about 3 days.

your three-day cleanse

In the following pages, you'll find my blueprint for a mind-clearing, soul-lifting, body-enlivening three-day reset.

As I mentioned earlier, this plan is for everyone: folks who are just getting started with juices and smoothies, juicing and blending pros, and those of you who love the taste of these drinks but sometimes find it challenging to stick with the habit. In the three days I've mapped out for you, you'll have a chance to ignite your love of clean nutrition. More important, you'll give your body the opportunity to soak in some easy-to-digest juices, blends, and meals. By the end of these three days, you should feel rejuvenated, focused, and inspired.

The point of this refresh is to restore—not to starve. Cleansing can actually be quite joyful. Fasting, on the other hand, can make you want to eat a sofa cushion slathered in butter. So with that in mind, I've given you two morning juices; a lunchtime blend; an afternoon juice, blend, or snack option; a healthy dinner; and a warm evening nut milk to savor. But if you find that you're hungry in spite of these options, don't hesitate to modify the plan and have a snack at any point. I've included a list of my ten favorite healthy snack options, which can all be enjoyed in addition to the options in the three-day plan. Lastly, make sure to drink plenty of water throughout each day.

To get started, use the grocery list provided to prep for your three-day adventure.

Then it's as easy as following along with the juices, smoothies, and meals listed. All of the recipes in bold are provided following the meal plan (they're listed right after the snacks).

During your three-day cleanse, you'll be taking a break from stimulating substances like coffee and alcohol. Don't worry; they'll be there for you when you're done—though you'll probably want to create a new relationship to them. Feel free to include herbal tea or green tea, if desired. You'll also step away from gluten and animal products, both of which can be irritating and taxing on your system. When we abruptly change our diets (like when we're cleansing) it's common to face some digestive disruption. Review my recommendations for constipation or loose stools (page 111) and all my self-care tips (pages 101–104). Epsom salt bath? Yup, it's got your name all over it!

Take some time to meditate, move your magnificent body, and reflect. Clear your calendar if possible (or at least pull back). Make space for your precious self. Juices, smoothies, and healthy foods are only part of the restorative process; in order to get the most benefit from this experience, you'll need to take care of both your body and spirit. At the end of this experience, you may be surprised at all the new ideas and ah-ha's that come rushing in as a result of some clean food and a clear head.

Drink up, rest up, and enjoy!

YOUR THREE-DAY CLEANSE

UPON RISING: Warm water with a squeeze of lemon and ginger. Remember also to drink plenty of water throughout the day.

8 A.M.: 8 to 10 ounces (1 serving) Classic Green Lemonade (page 127)

10:30 A.M.: 8 to 10 ounces (1 serving) Tummy Tamer (page 157)

1 P.M.: 8 to 10 ounces (1 serving) Easygoing Green Smoothie (page 199)

4 P.M.: 8 to 10 ounces (1 serving) Blueberry Lemon-Aid (page 163) and snack of choice (choose from list of snack options, page 313)

7 P.M.: Large salad with raw or gently steamed vegetables of choice, 2 tablespoons raw pumpkin seeds, ½ cup **Herbed Lentils** (page 300), and 3 tablespoons **Lemon Tahini Dressing** (page 308)

9 P.M.: 8 ounces Turmeric Milk (page 283), warmed

UPON RISING: Warm water with a squeeze of lemon and ginger. Remember also to drink plenty of water throughout the day.

8 A.M.: 8 to 10 ounces (1 serving) Rise 'n' Shine (page 173)

10:30 A.M.: 8 to 10 ounces (1 serving) Green Me Up (page 130)

1 P.M.: 8 to 10 ounces (1 serving) Inflammation Heavyweight (page 220)

4 P.M.: 8 to 10 ounces (1 serving) Savory Green Smoothie (page 206)

7 P.M.: 1 cup **Lemon Quinoa** (page 299) with 1 to 2 cups raw or steamed vegetables of choice, 2 tablespoons hemp seeds, and **Cilantro Lime Vinaigrette** (page 309)

9 P.M.: 8 ounces Chocolate Almond Milk (page 279), warmed

UPON RISING: Warm water with a squeeze of lemon and ginger. Remember also to drink plenty of water throughout the day.

8 A.M.: 8 to 10 ounces (1 serving) Pucker Up (page 177)

10:30 A.M.: 8 to 10 ounces (1 serving) Garden-in-a-Glass (page 142)

1 P.M.: 8 to 10 ounces (1 serving) Body Builder (page 219)

4 P.M.: 8 to 10 ounces (1 serving) Fatigue Fighter (page 193) and snack of choice (choose from list of snack options, page 313)

7 P.M.: 2 cups **Zucchini Noodles** (page 303), served raw or lightly sautéed in a teaspoon of olive oil, with ¼ cup **Cashew Cheese** (page 304), ½ cup **Herbed Lentils** (page 300), fresh chopped basil, and ⅓ cup **Raw Marinara** Sauce (page 305). Serve with extra steamed veggies if desired.

9 P.M.: 8 ounces Cashew Chai Milk (page 281), warmed

10

THE
THREE-DAY
CLEANSE
RECIPES

lemon quinoa

Yields Approximately 3 Cups

1 cup quinoa, dry

2 cups vegetable broth or water

1 tablespoon lemon juice

1 teaspoon lemon zest, grated

1 tablespoon olive oil or flax oil

Salt and pepper, to taste

2 tablespoons fresh parsley, leaves only, minced (optional)

1. Place the quinoa in a fine strainer and rinse it under cold water until the water runs clear.

2. Place the quinoa and broth in a medium pot. Bring the liquid to a boil. Cover and reduce heat to a simmer. Cook the quinoa for 20 minutes, or until all of the liquid is absorbed. Fluff the quinoa with a fork and allow it to rest for 15 minutes.

3. Stir the lemon juice and zest, olive oil, salt and pepper, and parsley into the quinoa. Serve. This will keep for up to five days, stored in an airtight container and refrigerated.

herbed lentils

1 cup green, black, or brown lentils, dried

1 clove garlic, minced

2½ cups vegetable broth or water

½ tablespoon fresh thyme, leaves only, minced
(or ½ teaspoon dried thyme)

2 tablespoons parsley, leaves only, minced
(or 1 tablespoon dried parsley)

1 tablespoon olive oil

1 tablespoon lemon juice

Salt and pepper, to taste

1   Place the lentils, garlic, and broth or water in a medium pot and bring them to a boil. Reduce the heat to a simmer and cover. Cook until the lentils have absorbed all of the liquid, approximately 20 to 30 minutes. If the lentils are still too firm after they've absorbed all of the liquid, you can add a little more water or broth until they're tender.

2   Allow the lentils to cool for 10 minutes. Toss the cooked lentils with the thyme, parsley, olive oil, lemon juice, and salt and pepper. Serve. This will keep for up to four days, stored in an airtight container and refrigerated.

almond ginger pate

Yields 1¼ Cups

1 cup almonds, soaked 8 hours

2 tablespoons lemon juice

1-inch piece ginger, peeled and grated

1 clove garlic, minced

1 tablespoon tamari or nama shoyu

1 tablespoon miso paste

½ cup carrots, grated (optional)

1   Place almonds in a food processor and process till they're coarsely ground.

2   With motor of the machine running, add ⅓ cup water in a thin stream, and then add the lemon juice, ginger, garlic, tamari, and miso. Stop the machine and check the texture; you want it to be very spreadable, but not so loose as to resemble a sauce. Continue processing until the mixture is smooth.

3   Pulse in the grated carrots, if using. This will keep for up to five days, stored in an airtight container and refrigerated.

zucchini noodles

2 large zucchini or summer squash, ends trimmed

1   Use one of the three methods below to create about 3 to 4 cups of fresh zucchini noodles. You can serve these raw, with a dressing or sauce, or sauté them with a teaspoon or two of olive oil till tender before enjoying them.

METHOD 1: Use a julienne peeler or the julienne blade of a mandolin to slice the zucchini lengthwise into long ribbons.

METHOD 2: Run a regular vegetable peeler along the length of your zucchini, pressing firmly. You'll create long noodle shapes.

METHOD 3: You can use a spiralizer to create super authentic zucchini noodles. (Spiralizers are fairly inexpensive and fun to use; my favorite is the Paderno spirooli, which retails for about $35.)

zucchini hemp hummus

Yields 1½ Cups

2 cups zucchini, peeled and roughly chopped

½ cup tahini

¼ cup shelled hemp seeds

3 tablespoons lemon juice

2 cloves garlic, minced

1 teaspoon cumin

Salt and pepper to taste

1   Blend all ingredients in a high-speed blender or food processor till smooth. If you use a food processor, you'll need to run the motor for a few minutes and stop and start the machine a few times in order to scrape the bowl down. Serve with crisp raw veggies, such as carrots, celery sticks, broccoli, cherry tomatoes, or cucumber slices. The zucchini hummus with keep in an airtight container in the fridge for up to three days.

tamari roasted chickpeas

2 cups cooked chickpeas, or one 16-ounce can chickpeas, rinsed

1 tablespoon olive oil

2 tablespoons balsamic vinegar

2 tablespoons tamari

2 teaspoons maple syrup

1   Preheat oven to 400 degrees Fahrenheit. Line a baking sheet with parchment paper.

2   Add all ingredients to a small mixing bowl and mix them well. Spread the mixture out onto the baking sheet.

3   Bake chickpea mixture for 25 to 30 minutes, or until it becomes crispy. Remove from the oven and flip the chickpeas around halfway through cooking. This will keep for up to one week, stored in an airtight container and refrigerated.

energy balls

1 cup almonds, walnuts, or cashews

¼ teaspoon sea salt

1 cup Medjool dates, pitted and tightly packed

1   Place the nuts and salt in the bowl of a food processor. Process until the ingredients are roughly ground.

2   Add the Medjool dates and continue processing until the ingredients look like a uniform meal. When you can squeeze some of the mixture in your hand and it sticks together easily, you're done.

3   Roll the mixture into balls 1 inch in diameter and refrigerate them for 30 minutes prior to serving. They will keep for up to two weeks, stored in an airtight container and refrigerated.

THREE-DAY CLEANSE SNACK OPTIONS

1 1 cup cucumber slices with ¼ cup **Zucchini Hemp Hummus** (page 307)

2 1 apple with 2 tablespoons almond butter

3 Small handful almonds and 4 dried, unsulphured apricots

4 8 to 10 ounces (1 serving) Savory Green Smoothie (page 206)

5 2 **Energy Balls** (page 312)

6 Celery sticks with ¼ cup **Almond Ginger Pate** (page 301)

7 1 banana, wrapped in a romaine leaf and spread with a tablespoon of peanut butter

8 ½ avocado, sliced and topped with lemon juice and a pinch of salt

9 ½ cup **Tamari Roasted Chickpeas** (page 311)

10 1 cup strawberries, sprinkled with 2 tablespoons shelled hemp seeds

GROCERY LIST FOR THE CLEANSE

PRODUCE & FRESH FOODS

- APPLES (5)
- AVOCADOS (2)
- BANANAS (3)
- BASIL (1 BUNCH)
- BEET (1)
- BELL PEPPER, YELLOW OR RED (1)
- BLUEBERRIES (1 PINT)
- BROCCOLI (1 STEM)
- CARROTS (7)
- CELERY (1 BUNCH, OR 8-10 STALKS)
- CHERRIES, FROZEN (ONE 4-OUNCE BAG)
- CHERRY TOMATOES (1 PINT) OR ROMA TOMATOES (3)
- CILANTRO (1 BUNCH)
- CUCUMBER (7)
- FENNEL (1 SMALL HEAD)
- GARLIC (1 HEAD)
- GINGER (1 PIECE, APPROXIMATELY 5-6 INCHES LONG)
- GRAPEFRUIT (2)

- GRAPES (1½ CUPS)
- KALE (1 BUNCH)
- LEMONS (5)
- LIMES (2)
- MANGO, FROZEN (ONE 8-OUNCE BAG)
- MEDJOOL DATES (10-12)
- MINT (1 BUNCH)
- NAVEL ORANGES (3)
- PARSLEY (1 BUNCH)
- PEARS (2)
- PINEAPPLE (1, OR 3 CUPS OF PINEAPPLE CHUNKS)
- ROMAINE (1 BUNCH, OR 12 LEAVES)
- SPINACH (1 BUNCH, OR 5 OUNCES BABY SPINACH)
- SWISS CHARD (1 BUNCH)
- THYME (1 BUNCH)
- TURMERIC ROOT (1 PIECE, APPROXIMATELY ½-INCH LONG)
- ZUCCHINI (3)

DAIRY ALTERNATIVES

- ALMOND MILK (56 OUNCES)
- COCONUT MILK (ONE 4-OUNCE CAN)
- NUTRITIONAL YEAST (SMALL OR LARGE FLAKE)

HERBS & SPICES

- CARDAMOM, GROUND
- CHILI FLAKES
- CINNAMON, GROUND
- CUMIN
- GINGER POWDER
- OREGANO, DRIED
- PARSLEY, DRIED
- THYME, DRIED
- TURMERIC POWDER

PANTRY GOODS

- ALMONDS (RAW)
- BALSAMIC VINEGAR
- CACAO POWDER
- CASHEWS (RAW)
- CHICKPEAS (ONE 16-OUNCE CAN)
- COCONUT WATER (16 OUNCES)
- GREEN, BLACK, OR BROWN LENTILS, DRY
- MAPLE SYRUP (OPTIONAL)
- MISO PASTE
- OLIVE OIL
- PEANUT BUTTER (ALL NATURAL)
- PUMPKIN SEEDS
- QUINOA, DRY
- SHELLED HEMP SEEDS
- SUN-DRIED TOMATOES (OIL PACKED OR DRY)
- TAHINI (RAW OR ROASTED)
- TAMARI
- VEGETABLE BROTH (2 QUARTS, OPTIONAL)

that's all, folks!

I hope you enjoy these recipes for years to come. Make them your own and share them with your friends and family. Take in the wisdom and use it as often as needed. I'm so very excited for your beaming future.

Oh, and I'd love to stay in touch and see your beautiful creations! Snap a pic of your juice or blend du jour and share it using #crazysexyjuice. I'm always running contests and giving away prizes. Who knows—perhaps you'll snag a sensational gift!

Once again, you can find me at Kriscarr.com and on social media—where I love sharing recipes, tips, inspiration, and pictures of my dogs. Come on over and join my lovely community. You'll meet lots of new friends and get encouraging messages from yours truly.

Big smooch and bottoms up to your awesomeness!

Peace & Veggies,

Kris

f Facebook www.facebook.com/KrisCarr.FanPage **Instagram** Crazysexykris

Twitter Kris_Carr **Pinterest** www.pinterest.com/CrazySexyKris/

INDEX

ACKNOWLEDGMENTS

I often save the best for last, but in this case I want to shine a big ole spotlight on the most important person to this project—my friend, recipe collaborator, and fellow nutrition junkie, Gena Hamshaw. Sister, we did it again. Thank you so much for all your hard work and dedication to this project. Without you, none of this fine goodness would be possible. Your testing and tweaking of all the recipes, your sound nutrition advice, and your brilliant edits were invaluable! You make the world a healthier place, dear one. Check out her magic and delicious recipes at choosingraw.com. I love you, lady!

To Jen Reilly, R.D., who fact-checked my work and taught me oodles about every fruit and veggie under the sun. Thank you for always helping me put the best information forward. I treasure you and your smart brain.

To my talented and caring editors, Patty Gift, Laura Gray, Sally Mason, and Karen Kelly, thank you for your insight, spot-on suggestions, crazy fixes when I was out of solutions, and all the creativity you each breathed into this book. Thanks too for keeping me calm and creating time where there wasn't any.

To Reid Tracy and Patty Gift for saying yes to this juicy goodness and for always giving me creative space and support. I'm endlessly grateful for your belief in me.

To Brian (my hubby), thank you for always reading (and editing!) my work and for challenging me when you know I can do better. You're the best partner in life and creativity a gal could ever ask for. And, oh my goodness, thank you for wearing frilly aprons, cleaning the juicer a thousand times, and tasting each and every recipe. You're a champ!

To my pal Jan Mann, this book's nanny! Thank you for helping me shop, prep, chop, juice, blend, and taste test each of these fabulous elixirs every Tuesday and Thursday for months! You are a fabulous sous chef, and so many of your ah-ha's and ooh-la-la's made it into the manuscript. Bless you!

To Kate Lewis for your beautiful, whimsical, clever photography. I asked you to tell stories with each picture and you nailed it. Thank you so much for capturing my vision and expanding my style.

To Bill Miles for your wonderful cover. Dude, you're a genius, and you're the only one who makes me feel comfortable in front of the camera. Oh, and thank you for also being my Photoshop orthodontist and hairdresser—cream rinse!

To Karla Baker for your badass designs and creative fire. Thank you for bringing your beautiful talent and spirit to my vision. You've been on this journey with me since my first book, and I really appreciate how you allow me to grow in each project. I love all our book designs, but I gotta say, I might love this one best! It's gorgeous, like you.

To my wonderful team at Crazy Sexy Wellness—Corinne Bowen, Ashley Zink, Maria Mooney, and Jessica Kennedy. Ladies, I couldn't do it without you. Thank you for your creative brilliance and dedication, and for caring about the world and all the animals. I am grateful for each of you every day.

ABOUT THE AUTHOR

Kris Carr is a multi-week *New York Times* best-selling author, speaker, and wellness activist. She is the subject and director of the documentary *Crazy Sexy Cancer*, which premiered at the SXSW Film Festival and aired on TLC, The Discovery Channel, and The Oprah Winfrey Network. Kris is also the author of the award-winning Crazy Sexy book series. Her latest books, *Crazy Sexy Diet* and *Crazy Sexy Kitchen*, will change the way you live, love, and eat! Kris regularly lectures at hospitals, wellness centers, corporations such as Whole Foods, and Harvard University. Named a "new role model" by the *New York Times*, she has been featured in *Glamour*, *Vanity Fair*, *Scientific American*, *Success*, *Forbes*, *People*, *Good Morning America*, the *Today* show, *CBS Evening News*, *Access Hollywood*, *The Doctors*, *Super Soul Sunday*, and *The Oprah Winfrey Show*. As an irreverent foot soldier in the fight against disease, Kris inspires countless people to take charge of their health and happiness by adopting a plant-passionate diet, self-care practices, and learning to live and love like they really mean it. In Oprah's words, "Kris Carr's riveting journey started a revolution." Visit her at Kriscarr.com.

We hope you enjoyed this Hay House book. If you'd like to receive our online catalog featuring additional information on Hay House books and products, or if you'd like to find out more about the Hay Foundation, please contact:

Hay House, Inc., P.O. Box 5100, Carlsbad, CA 92018-5100
(760) 431-7695 or (800) 654-5126
(760) 431-6948 (fax) or (800) 650-5115 (fax)
www.hayhouse.com® • www.hayfoundation.org

Published and distributed in Australia by: Hay House Australia Pty. Ltd., 18/36 Ralph St., Alexandria NSW 2015 • Phone: 612-9669-4299 Fax: 612-9669-4144 • www.hayhouse.com.au

Published and distributed in the United Kingdom by: Hay House UK, Ltd., Astley House, 33 Notting Hill Gate, London W11 3JQ • Phone: 44-20-3675-2450 Fax: 44-20-3675-2451 • www.hayhouse.co.uk

Published and distributed in the Republic of South Africa by: Hay House SA (Pty.), Ltd., P.O. Box 990, Witkoppen 2068 • info@hayhouse.co.za • www.hayhouse.co.za

Published in India by: Hay House Publishers India, Muskaan Complex, Plot No. 3, B-2, Vasant Kunj, New Delhi 110 070 • Phone: 91-11-4176-1620 Fax: 91-11-4176-1630 • www.hayhouse.co.in

Distributed in Canada by: Raincoast Books, 2440 Viking Way, Richmond, B.C. V6V 1N2 • Phone: 1-800-663-5714 • Fax: 1-800-565-3770 • www.raincoast.com

Take Your Soul on a Vacation

Visit www.HealYourLife.com® to regroup, recharge, and reconnect with your own magnificence. Featuring blogs, mind-body-spirit news, and life-changing wisdom from Louise Hay and friends.

Visit www.HealYourLife.com today!